Routledge Revivals

International Studies
Volume 2

First published in 1931, this book is the second of a three volume set which focuses on medical work, and in particular, public administration in relation to the prevention of disease. This volume focuses on the medical circumstances of Belgium, France, Italy, Jugo-Slavia, Hungary, Poland and Czecho-Slovakia. It shows that many of these countries have gone beyond most others in the socialization of medicine, in several ways.

T0139226

International Studies
Volume 2
Prevention and Treatment of Disease

Sir Arthur Newsholme

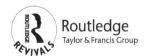

Routledge
Taylor & Francis Group

First published in 1931
by George Allen & Unwin

This edition first published in 2015 by Routledge
2 Park Square, Milton Park, Abingdon, Oxon, OX14 4RN
and by Routledge
711 Third Avenue, New York, NY 10017

Routledge is an imprint of the Taylor & Francis Group, an informa business

Publisher's Note
The publisher has gone to great lengths to ensure the quality of this reprint but
points out that some imperfections in the original copies may be apparent.

Disclaimer
The publisher has made every effort to trace copyright holders and welcomes
correspondence from those they have been unable to contact.

A Library of Congress record exists under LC control number: 32001245

ISBN 13: 978-1-138-91267-0 (hbk)
ISBN 13: 978-1-315-69183-1 (ebk)
ISBN 13: 978-1-138-91269-4 (pbk)

INTERNATIONAL STUDIES

ON THE RELATION BETWEEN THE

PRIVATE & OFFICIAL PRACTICE *of* MEDICINE

WITH SPECIAL REFERENCE TO

THE PREVENTION OF DISEASE

conducted for

THE MILBANK MEMORIAL FUND

by

SIR ARTHUR NEWSHOLME, K.C.B., M.D., F.R.C.P.

Volume Two

BELGIUM, FRANCE, ITALY
JUGO-SLAVIA, HUNGARY, POLAND
CZECHO-SLOVAKIA

LONDON: GEORGE ALLEN & UNWIN LTD
BALTIMORE: WILLIAMS & WILKINS CO

FIRST PUBLISHED IN 1931

FOREWORD

ON BEHALF OF THE MILBANK MEMORIAL FUND

ONE of the major problems in present-day public health administration is that of ascertaining the proper sphere of the private physician in the field of public health. Upon a number of occasions during the past few years this matter has been earnestly discussed by private physicians and public health administrators in joint assemblies arranged for the purpose, and some progress has been made in indicating what should be the relationship between private medicine and public health to ensure co-operative service in conserving the health of the public.

During the past seven years the Directors of the Milbank Memorial Fund have had occasion to consider this problem very seriously, in connection with the opposition of some members of the medical profession to certain phases of the public health work, which the Milbank Memorial Fund helped to inaugurate in one locality as a part of its participation in the New York State Health Demonstrations. This opposition led the Fund to re-examine the initial tenets upon which its participation in the health demonstrations was based, in order to make sure that its philanthropic service in the field of public health was not such as would in any way embarrass or impede fulfilment of the legitimate professional aspirations of the private medical practitioner. Finding in the history of public health development in the United States few precedents to guide them, the Directors decided to arrange for an international investigation to be made objectively and without bias, the purpose of the study being to throw light on the relationship in different countries between the fields of activity of private practising physicians and of physicians and laymen engaged in public health work. It was felt that studies of what was being done elsewhere in public health might be valuable in indicating not only solutions of difficult problems, particularly affecting the relation between private physicians and physicians engaged in public health work, but specifically in showing how the co-operative services of private physicians may be utilised to the highest advantage by public authorities. Such problems have arisen whenever preventive medicine has become in part clinical in character.

In various countries medical treatment of the poorer members of the community is provided apart from private medical practice:

1. By the Poor Law authorities, for the destitute;
2. By voluntary organisations, in hospitals, dispensaries, and similar institutions, for those who are destitute in the sense of not being able to pay for specially skilled help;
3. Under public insurance schemes, which may be limited to medical aid or may also give financial assistance, and in which the State and the employer are, or may be, partially responsible, as well as the beneficiary;
4. By public health authorities, given at the expense of the taxpayer, as, for instance, in fever and smallpox hospitals and in sanatoria for tuberculosis, in venereal disease clinics, and to a smaller extent in maternity and infant consultation centres; and
5. By school or public health authorities in school clinics, at which eye defects, skin complaints, adenoids and tonsils, dental caries and other defects, are treated either gratuitously or at a small cost proportionate to the resources of the patient.

In different countries the activities under these and allied headings vary enormously. The public increasingly realises that each member of the community must have prompt and adequate medical care. By this means protracted illness can be avoided, which in itself is a great public health gain; subsequent crops of such diseases as tuberculosis and the venereal diseases can be prevented; and the general standard of health and efficiency of the community can be raised.

As public health becomes more advanced and personal hygiene forms an increasing part of it, the stimulus to provide medical services either through voluntary or official organisations increases, and the delicacy of the relation between private medical practitioners and voluntary and official organisations becomes accentuated.

Hitherto, most countries have evolved measures for reaching their hygienic objective only as each pressing need has emerged. There has been irregular and unbalanced progress, or stagnation has continued when opposition has been severe. The different countries have not learned adequately from each other; and at the present time, except as regards insurance schemes in England and Germany, but little international information of an accurate and authentic character is available for the medical profession and for social workers.

For the reasons incompletely set forth above, the Directors of the Milbank Memorial Fund, in the summer of 1928, secured the services of Sir Arthur Newsholme, M.D., K.C.B., former chief medical officer of the Local Government Board of England and Wales, and lecturer on public health administration, School of Hygiene and Public Health, the Johns Hopkins University, to make on their behalf: (1) an objective study of what is being done in the treatment as well as in the prevention of disease in the chief European countries, including Great Britain and Ireland; and (2) an impartial study of the philosophy of the subject, with the hope that therefrom there will emerge further possibilities of action for the public good, and at the same time not inimical to the real interests of the medical profession. The Directors of the Milbank Memorial Fund are confident that the two interests are essentially identical; but they believe it important to base any conclusions and recommendations that may be reached on the foundation of a wide and international investigation, which has been objective in character. In securing the services of Sir Arthur Newsholme to make the inquiries included in this series, the Milbank Directors had confidence that his long experience with the problems discussed in the studies and his familiarity with conditions both in England and in America qualified him to present an accurate account in perspective of the pitfalls and triumphs of preventive medicine and public health administration in the different countries concerned. It is understood, of course, that the Directors of the Milbank Memorial Fund in submitting herewith the findings of Sir Arthur Newsholme's international investigation do not commit the Fund to endorse his views in any respect or to approve the methods of public health work described. It is to be remembered that the essence of the investigation is to throw light on the relationship in different countries between practising physicians on the one hand, and physicians and authorities in public health work on the other hand; and this consideration explains the choice of subjects discussed in each chapter, which are selected as best illustrating this main problem.

JOHN A. KINGSBURY
Secretary

PREFACE TO VOLUME TWO

THIS volume, as already indicated by Mr. Kingsbury in his introduction contributed on behalf of the Milbank Memorial Fund, is second of three volumes describing the circumstances of medical work in a number of European countries as related to public administration, local and national, when this concerns itself with direct measures for the prevention or treatment of disease.

The investigation, the results of which for a group of countries are here summarised, was undertaken to obtain a record of observed facts; and although here and there reflections on these facts have been made, the present and its companion volumes maintain this limitation. In an independent volume general problems are considered.

Evidently a survey of every branch of curative and preventive medicine is beyond the power of any single investigator, unless years were devoted to it, which would make the observations out of date before they were published. It has been necessary, therefore, to proceed by sampling these medical activities, selecting those which are typical or exceptional, and which are specially instructive to the workers engaged in medical administration or in private medical practice, who desire to have the light of experience in other fields thrown on their own problems.

Although the survey, as I have made it, is only partial, much perhaps is gained from the fact that the survey has been made by one person only, and that the facts and observations embodied in it are thus fairly comparable. It may be added that the writer's familiarity for several decades with the task of selecting and assessing the salient features in actual public health problems has made his present task less laborious than it would otherwise have been, and has enabled him to select subjects concerning which an interchange of experience is most important.

My earliest inquiries in this investigation soon revealed the fact that in nearly every country visited by me almost identical difficulties were being experienced, some in their initial and others in their later stages; and ere long it became evident that these difficulties centred around certain specific medical problems. These are methods of medical attendance on the poor, the provision of hospital treatment and consultative facilities for the sick, the medical phase of sickness insurance, and the special problems of maternity and child welfare work, of school medical work, and of work for the treatment and prevention of tuberculosis and venereal diseases. In nearly every country it is concerning these problems that the "snags" of private medical practice in relation to the organised community recur and recur; and, although other aspects of medical work are not ignored when points of interest emerge, it is to the study of the practice in regard to the above-mentioned problems that the following pages are chiefly devoted.

In order to understand the medical problems in each country studied, it has been found necessary to outline the governmental methods of the country concerned. Without this the administrative details of medical work would lose much of their significance.

In the present volume the medical circumstances of Belgium, France, Italy, Jugo-Slavia, Hungary, Poland and Czecho-Slovakia are placed under review—some in considerable detail, others more sketchily. Some of these countries have gone farther than most other countries in the socialisation of medicine in one or another respect; and a study of the details of this movement has important bearings on the general problems behind the present investigation.

These general problems will be discussed in a separate volume, in which the experience in the different countries studied will be compared, and an attempt will be made to derive some general principles of action from the survey embodied in the preceding volumes.

Special attention, meanwhile, may be drawn to the paragraphs in the chapter on France, in which the medico-political problems of tuberculosis dispensaries and the new system of national sickness insurance are set out in some detail in their bearing on confidential private medical practice.

It should be added that the contents of each chapter in this volume have been carefully revised in each instance by an important medical official of the country concerned. Although in each chapter I have expressed my indebtedness to the chief officials concerned, I must here more generally voice my gratitude for unsparing help and corrections, which enable me with confidence to pass the following pages for the press. If any mistakes have been made, I am personally responsible.

ARTHUR NEWSHOLME

February 1931

TABLE OF CONTENTS

FRANCE (*continued*)

CHAPTER III

ITALY   124

INTERNATIONAL STUDIES

CHAPTER I

BELGIUM[1]

PRELIMINARY SUMMARY

Belgium presents interesting features in its medico-social arrangements.

It is rather densely populated, largely industrial, and its people are very frugal. Its alcoholic problem has been greatly improved since the Great War. Owing to acute religious and political differences, its numerous medico-social activities are much subdivided; they are largely subsidised by the State, with relatively light governmental restrictions.

School medical work is scantily developed. A large amount of child welfare work is done by voluntary agencies. Tuberculosis work similarly is voluntarily organised. Anti-venereal work, in which the active co-operation of private physicians has been obtained, has achieved much success.

The medical profession is organised into medical syndicates, which make it an essential condition of forthcoming compulsory sickness insurance that the doctor shall be paid in each case for actual work done.

A high proportion of the wage-earning population are already insured against sickness in voluntary societies, and in some of these the conditions of medical employment are unsatisfactory.

From the point of view of public medical work, Belgium has travelled much farther than France, but is possessed by the same determination as its southern neighbour (see pages 90 *et seq.*) to prevent the doctor from being involved in the speculative risks involved in any capitation arrangement of payment per insured person.

---

[1] Date of investigation, May 1930.

GENERAL OBSERVATIONS

In visiting Belgium one could not fail to be impressed by the bustling activity, the small amount of unemployment up to the date of writing, and the optimism characterising its people in present circumstances. Belgium, the breach of whose internationally pledged neutrality was a determining factor of the World War, was overrun early in the war by Germans. Its population was thus put in large measure *hors de combat*, and relatively few of its men were killed. Some share of the present resilience of the Belgians may be due to the fact that in the European holocaust only a relatively small part of its virile population was sacrificed.

But although Belgium suffered less in, and has recovered more completely after, the war than other European countries, its standard of living is lower than that of English-speaking countries. Wages are low, and the cost of living does not completely correspond to the wages; and the social and medical needs of the country have to be met in accordance with this basic fact.

Belgium has a population of about 7 millions, distributed in nine provinces which lie between The Netherlands, Prussia, France, and the North Sea.

Its people are commonly bilingual, Flemish and Walloon or French, the Flemish outnumbering the Walloon population by about a million. The French population is predominantly industrial, and the Flemish predominantly agricultural and horticultural, though this distinction is becoming less marked.

In the French provinces the population is less strictly Roman Catholic than in the Flemish section.

The birth-rate in Belgium in 1927 was 18·3 per 1,000 of population; prior to the war it had stood between 19 and 20 for some thirty years. It varies considerably in different parts of Belgium, though not apparently in accordance with the number who nominally adhere to the Roman Catholic teaching on conception-control. Since the war a law has been enacted against conception-control, but it is doubtful if it is effective. A recent work by a Catholic priest, Père

Lemaire, is entitled *La Wallonie qui meurt*. Some midwives are said to be largely responsible for the production of abortion, which is stated to be frequent.

As already stated, there is, hitherto, very little unemployment in Belgium, though an impending increase is anticipated. The main industries have been combined in large associations, and thus it is claimed increased efficiency and economy of effort have been secured. Industries in the hands of private individuals are exceptional. In agriculture also the practice of combined buying of seeds and combined selling of produce prevails. Owing to the dearth of workers, many Poles and Italians have come into Belgium since the war, and are employed in its coal-mines and elsewhere. A farm labourer is paid about 30 francs a day, and an industrial worker may obtain as much as 70 francs. (£1 sterling = 175 Belgian francs, or approximately $5.) This may be exceptional: a skilled municipal workman in Brussels receives 55 francs.

The position of Belgium as regards alcoholic consumption has greatly improved. Its beer is light, and spirits, including liqueurs, are not allowed to be served to customers in restaurants and hotels. No spirituous drink can be bought in quantity below 2 litres (4 pints). The result is that for the poorer people the drinking of spirits is negligible in amount. This is a by-product of the Great War; but it has been endorsed by the electorate, the majority of whom are socialist. Prior to the war, absenteeism from work on Mondays after Sunday's drinking was common. The drinking of wine also has decreased since the war; and I am assured that alcoholism as a disease has almost disappeared, like the Monday absenteeism of workers.

Another important social reform may be mentioned in passing. In every chief prison there is an *anthropological service*. Every prisoner detained more than six months or detained for a second time is examined completely. Prisoners are then classified and are drafted according to the findings to insane asylums, tuberculosis sanatoria, colonies for feeble-minded and epileptics, etc., or they are placed on parole. Under a new law recidivists can be segregated almost indefinitely. The same law provides for psychological and psychiatric examination of the offender before trial. It thus appears that important advance has been made in the individualisation and scientific reform of penal justice.

GOVERNMENT

The government of Belgium is that of a constitutional monarchy. No act of the King is effective unless counter-signed by one of his Ministers.

There are ten Ministers, and the same number of Government Departments. Of these, four—the Ministers of the Interior, of Labour and of Social Insurance, of Justice, and of Education—are concerned with the subject of this investigation.

There are two Houses in the legislature, the Senate and the Chamber of Representatives. All elections for the latter are on the principle of universal suffrage for all men and women over 21 years of age. The principle of proportional representation is followed. The majority of the senators are chosen by universal suffrage; some are chosen by the provincial councils, on the basis of one for 200,000 inhabitants; and a further proportion is chosen by the Senate itself.

LOCAL ADMINISTRATION

The nine provinces of Belgium contain 41 arrondisse-ments and 2,672 communes. The communes vary in popula-tion from 100 to 300,000. Brussels itself consists of eight larger and some smaller communes, having almost com-pletely independent health administration.

Each of the nine provinces has a salaried governor, whose appointment is political. The provincial council is con-cerned with the upkeep of roads, control of epidemics, and maintenance of certain institutions.

Each communal council consists of from seven to forty-five members elected by the male population for six years, on the basis of proportional representation. The members are unpaid, except the aldermen.

The local burgomaster is appointed by the King. He is also registrar (*officier de l'état civil*) and chief of the Police. He is, in large measure, an uncontrolled autocrat.

The executive committee of the communal council is known as the Collège des Bourgmestres et Echevins. Its aldermen are elected from the communal council for six years, and they are salaried.

In every commune there is a Commission d'Assistance appointed by the communal or municipal council. This commission manages the local hospitals, dispensaries, and asylums; gives monetary relief to the destitute, and organises their medical treatment. Smaller communes send their patients to hospitals owned by other municipalities, or to private hospitals, paying a charge, which is fixed by the Government. A Consultative Council attached to the Ministry of Justice (*Conseil Supérieur de la bienfaisance*) in 1919–21 made an official inquiry into the conditions of poor relief. The inquiry showed that throughout Belgium, and especially in the smaller communes, the poor law medical service lacked resources and organisation. Many of the smaller residential institutions for the old and sick almost entirely lacked medical equipment. Evidently, as in England not many years ago, and still in some areas, reforms are needed. There are about 280 hospitals in Belgium, of which 164 are public and 116 private. These have a bed-capacity of 17,000. Insane asylums are not included in this enumeration.

CENTRAL ADMINISTRATION

In my inquiry into this I received valuable guidance from Dr. Timbal, the Directeur Général de l'Administration de l'Hygiène.

A central staff of medical and other technical inspectors are employed for the general supervision of health matters. The medical inspectors act to some extent as provincial medical officers of health.

There are two chief divisions of central administration concerned respectively with vital statistics and with public health.

The central administration of public assistance is at the Ministry of Justice. It concerns itself with poor law supervision, the insane, cripples, blind, deaf-mutes, and the mentally deficient.

The Ministry of Labour has the direction of industrial hygiene, inspection of work-places, and medical services for employed persons in mutual sickness insurance societies (mutualités).

This separation of functions is not very conducive to efficiency, and especially so as the central authorities have no control over the activity or inactivity of municipalities, except in so far as they give grants-in-aid.

Medical administration, both locally and centrally, is largely helped by advisory and voluntary committees. Among these advisory bodies are the Royal Academy of Medicine, the Higher Council of Hygiene, a Pharmacopœal Commission, Commissioners on Cancer, Commissioners on the supervision of production of vaccines, etc.

There are, in addition, the Red Cross of Belgium, the Central Office for the Study of Alcoholism, and the National Society for the Protection of Infancy (L'Œuvre Nationale de l'Enfance).

Each province has from one to three provincial medical commissions, which exercise supervision over medical practitioners, midwives, and dentists; and there are provincial health inspectors. The medical members of the commission are nominated by the physicians and pharmacists of the province. In most of the provinces the Provincial Government has created a bacteriological institute in which are made gratuitous analyses of blood, urine, etc., and from which are supplied sera and vaccines. Some of these institutes have played an important part in the hygienic movement against tuberculosis, ankylostomiasis, etc. The province of Hainaut has a museum of hygiene for the general public.

The work of local authorities (provincial and communal) is confined in the main to ordinary sanitary work, and does not include special measures for the treatment and prevention of tuberculosis or for the protection of infancy. These activities, as will shortly be seen, are entrusted to special *ad hoc* organisations, perhaps necessitated by acute political and religious differences. Although this segregation of special work, in my view, does not permit of the best possible results, much valuable work is being carried out by these special organisations (as also by the Ligue Nationale Belge contre le Péril Vénérien), and it may be that this separation of duties is fitted to the present stage of development of public health in Belgium.

The Red Cross has organised a transportation service for the sick and wounded, and a first-class service for streets, mines, etc.

It has also embarked on other activities. In Brussels it has a health centre (child welfare, tuberculosis, venereal disease, and mental hygiene dispensaries). It has several mental hygiene dispensaries. Under its auspices a National Health Council has been formed. This is not, I am informed, very active.

We need not enumerate the ordinary activities of public health, local and central, authorities, as they do not present any noteworthy feature. The work of these authorities is not aided by adequate co-ordination between different authorities. Brussels itself comprises eight separate local governmental bodies, each of these in the main independent of the others; and within these eight communes, as in communes throughout Belgium, the character of local administration varies greatly in accordance with local politics—whether Catholic, Liberal, or Socialist—and with financial conditions.

This acute separation of political and religious interests pervades all public affairs. In a given commune there may be separate child welfare centres for each of these three sections, and there may be an additional "Neutral" centre.

Similar divisions characterise Red Cross and tuberculosis

activities; all of these receiving subsidies from the Government. An identical remark applies to sickness insurance in mutualités. Hospital provision suffers to a less extent from divisions in accordance with religious beliefs.

The Medical and Allied Professions

In 1927 there were in Belgium—

5,232 medical practitioners, or one for 1,520 inhabitants;
2,686 midwives, or one for 2,950 inhabitants;
2,080 pharmacists, or one for 3,810 inhabitants;
579 dentists, or one for 13,690 inhabitants.

The proportion of doctors varies greatly in the different provinces. In Antwerp they are two and a half times as many as the midwives; in Luxembourg midwives and doctors are equal in number; and in Limbourg midwives are somewhat more numerous than doctors.

Some of the conditions of medical practice are detailed in the section relating to mutualités. The organised medical profession holds strongly to the view that in contracts for insurance the medical profession should be outside the terms of any contract on an insurance basis, and be paid an agreed sum for each medical "act", whether consultation or visit.

Practice of Midwives

Midwives are partially supervised by the Provincial Health Commissions and to a limited extent by medical inspectors of the Government.

They are supposed not to be allowed to practise without a diploma, which is given after a three-years' course of training, but, in fact, "handy-women" practise midwifery on a considerable scale. In the training-school it is required that each group of ten pupils shall have attended annually during her three years' training at least fifty confinements. Midwives must have undergone prior training for two years as a nurse. The details of the course of training both for nurses and midwives are given in full in the official regulations.

The practice of the midwife is regulated. She is limited to attending on normal parturition. She may only administer ergot after delivery, and laudanum only while awaiting a doctor in a case of threatened abortion. In all abnormal cases she must call in a doctor.

A recent circular has been issued by La Commission Médicale Provinciale of Gand to midwives which illustrates the rigid attitude of the medical profession and the general character of the instruction given to midwives. In this circular the midwife is warned against undertaking medical functions, and it is particularly enjoined that she should not give advice to mothers on wasting or diarrhœa in infants. She may weigh babies, but must not give advice on the method of feeding them. In particular she must not advise on swollen legs in expectant mothers. When she is engaged by the mother for a confinement she may diagnose the presentation and examine the urine, but must refer the case to a doctor if anything abnormal is found. If it is objected that the patient thus referred is unlikely to return to the midwife, it is argued that she will return as soon as conditions become normal. (See *Fédération Méd. Belge, Bulletin Official*, March 1929.)

The usual fee given to a midwife is 300 francs, to a doctor the minimum fee is 500 francs.

The proportion of confinements attended by midwives varies from 25 to 50 per cent. of the total births.

PUERPERAL MORTALITY

In the three years 1925–27 the recorded puerperal death-rate per 1,000 live-births was in—

1925 ..	..	..	..	5·3
1926 ..	..	..	..	6·62
1927 ..	..	..	..	5·72

of which nearly 54 per cent. was recorded as due to sepsis, and the rest to other accidents of childbirth and pregnancy. In this connection the frequency of abortion may be recalled. The puerperal death-rate is much higher than that of Denmark and Holland; and it is unlikely that differences in certification and classification of deaths can account for more than a small proportion of this excess. Indeed, it seems likely that the certification of puerperal mortality in Belgium is not quite complete, as death-certification is not infrequently non-medical.

L'ŒUVRE NATIONALE DE L'ENFANCE

This body, which is referred to below as O.N.E., is the agency which has a monopoly of child welfare work in Belgium.

The past history of such work in Belgium does not differ greatly from that in other countries. The first Consultation de Nourissons (Consultations for Infants) was started in 1897, and crèches[1] were then already in existence. A national league for co-ordinating measures for the protection of infancy was constituted in 1903; and from 1908 onwards the Government subsidised some of this work. In 1914 there were in Belgium seventy such consultations.

During the war special efforts were made, especially for the feeding of infants and young children, and when the armistice came there were 768 consultations and 473 maternal cantines, nearly as many cantines for weakly children, and over 2,000 centres for school meals. In the inauguration and support of this work American charity and American doctors bore a noble part.

After the war, work for the protection of infants and the promotion of child hygiene was nationalised under the title given at the head of this section by a law passed September 5, 1919. The O.N.E. thus has become an official body, subsidised almost to the full extent of its expenses by the Government, but under the management of a voluntary organisation.

There is first of all a Conseil Supérieur to direct the work. This consists of at least forty members, nominated for five

[1] As the terms crèche, day nursery, and nursery school are frequently used in the text, it may be stated here that all three are intended to supplement maternal care for children under school age. The two first have an almost identical meaning. In a nursery school more formal instruction is initiated. Cantines are stations for providing meals, gratuitously or for a small payment.

years, in the first instance by the King, and subsequently by the council itself, as vacancies occur.

This council regulates the local activities of all local committees of the O.N.E. in their work of initiating Consultations de Nourissons. The cost of each local consultation is borne to the extent of—

Half by the State,
Quarter by the province, and
Quarter by the commune.

As a rule there are no voluntary subscriptions. A new consultation may be demanded by any twenty mothers or future mothers, and a local committee can then be organised for this purpose. This has often led to the formation of multiple consultations, representing local political or religious leanings; and there appears to be no effective machinery to prevent this unnecessary redundance of effort, though the taxpayers must pay its cost.

The doctor's fee for attendance is 25–30 francs (175 francs = £1), with an additional 50 centimes for each baby seen up to fifty.

A local practitioner is appointed for this work, and usually no friction appears to arise with other practitioners. Sometimes there is a rota of doctors, but in this case it is arranged that parents always bring their children to see the same doctor.

No treatment is given as a rule. Most centres have visiting nurses attached to them. These attend and weigh the babies and give simple advice, and the doctor may see all or only certain cases. If there is no visiting nurse, then the local midwife is asked to undertake the home visiting. In such a case the midwife must give up her midwifery work, so as not to compete with other midwives.

Good attendances are secured at the consultations, and often these are continued in the second year of life.

The O.N.E. has also organised 266 prenatal consultations, the more complete of these being annexed to maternity hospitals, polyclinics, etc. These are not generally regarded by the mothers as necessary; and similarly home visitation of children attending infant consultations is far from being general in all parts of the country.

At one centre in Brussels I saw some extremely good consultation work, and the forms in use for recording familial and personal data were excellent. The same forms are in use at all consultations of the O.N.E. At this particular centre some treatment was given to sick children, including mercurial inunctions in cases of congenital syphilis. Owing to the poverty of the parents there appears to be no difficulty with private practitioners.

Crèches are included in the work of the O.N.E. One seen by me at Schaerbeck was most sumptuous and complete in its arrangements for about 200 children under two years old. There is much female industrial work, and the provision of crèches appears to be unavoidable. When measles becomes epidemic the crèche necessarily becomes a danger to young child life.

Other activities of the O.N.E. are not detailed, as they have little bearing on the relation between private doctors and the organisation. My thanks are accorded to M. Belge, the general secretary, and to Mademoiselle Nevejean, of the O.N.E., who gave me every facility in my inquiries.

SCHOOL MEDICAL WORK

This exists to a limited extent. Every commune is required by an enactment of 1921 to arrange for an examination of each pupil on his admission to the free schools of the State and for a monthly visit of a medical inspector to each school.

School medical inspectors are usually elected from among local medical practitioners by the communal council. These may also inspect the children in parochial (religious) schools, but are not permitted to control any of the arrangements for action. In most communes the service is still in its infancy, but in some good work is done. Dr. Nobert Ensch, the medical officer of health of Schaerbeck, a division of Brussels, gave me much valuable information as to his important work which has continued for many years in this borough. To him I am also indebted for valuable help in other respects. He has twelve schools under his supervision, with some 5,000 scholars, and he holds school consultations at two centres. Special cases are sent to a dentist, oculist, or throat specialist. The Government enacts that the work shall be done, but it is paid for entirely by the municipality, and consequently the work varies in amount and in quality according to the degree of enlightenment and the financial circumstances of each commune. In socialistic centres there is usually exceptional activity in health work, including school work.

A recent illustration may be given of a local effort towards an improved school medical service. In one of the progressive municipalities of Greater Brussels there were recently fifteen school doctors, whose efficiency was described to me as nearly nil. The municipality removed these from office and replaced them by a whole-time medical officer. The dismissed doctors appealed to the Collège des Médecins, but their record was considered so unsatisfactory that the Collège refrained from intervention.

ANTI-TUBERCULOSIS WORK

L'Association Nationale contre la Tuberculose and *La Ligue Nationale contre la Tuberculose* have divided between them Belgian work for the control of tuberculosis, the former dealing with establishments for its care, and the latter with general prophylaxis, centring around dispensaries; but recently the two organisations have been merged. In addition, there is a society for the scientific study of tuberculosis, and a special society dealing with the protection of infants against tuberculosis. The last-named undertakes on a limited scale to place suitably from birth infants born of tuberculous parents until the risk of infection is gone.

The two first-named are national organisations, and receive State subsidies for their work; and on their co-operation depends the indispensable liaison between the complementary preventive measures undertaken by them.

The league was created in 1898, a committee nominated by the Royal Society of Medicine being appointed, with a small grant for the costs of administration. The Director of the Central Committee directs its general work, and general supervision is exercised over the branches throughout Belgium.

In 1911 private generosity provided 75 per cent., the provinces and communes 22 per cent., and the Government 3 per cent. of the funds expended.

During the war help was obtained from the Comité National de Secours et d'Alimentation; and after the war the Government took its place, and now the Government and the Central Committee supply the greater part of the funds for local work. The dispensaries receive 70 per cent. of their expenses, apart from any funds spent on material relief.

The Government leaves to the league its autonomy and independence of work, only reserving control over the use made of the funds which it subscribes to the league.

Every dispensary has a visiting nurse, who sees patients at their homes.

It is unnecessary to describe in detail the work of sanatoria and allied institutions. After the war a capital sum of eleven million francs was subscribed by private charity, by banks, and by industrial firms for the erection of these institutions. Patients from mutualités and others are received at a charge of 23·50 francs per diem. If the patient cannot pay this the municipality may do so. The Government pays 2·50 francs per diem for every patient at a sanatorium or hospital, and subscribes 5,000 francs per bed towards the construction of new institutions. In connection with the hundredth anniversary of the Independence of Belgium the Government has decided to give a hundred million francs for the anti-tuberculosis movement.

Tuberculosis in 1910–13 caused a death-rate in Belgium of 1·6 per 1,000. In 1922 this had become 1·48, and in 1923 it was 1·06.

During 1928 the consultations at the dispensaries of the league numbered 171,678, of which 91,878 were for young children. The number of new patients was 19,408, of whom 11,825 were found to be tuberculous.

Of the patients in that year, 1886 were relegated for institutional treatment in sanatoria, and 2,309 in hospitals.

The physicians attached to these dispensaries number 195. These held 11,184 clinics during the year, and examined 98,174 persons clinically: 9,458 radiographic examinations were made.

Patients are treated at the dispensaries, and private physicians are engaged. There is said to be little difficulty with doctors in private practice.

It will be noted that in anti-tuberculosis work, as in infant welfare work, the State and local authorities take no direct part. They subscribe, but the actual work is undertaken by committees, central and local, which are not representative, in the sense of being elected either by the people or by the members of these authorities.

ANTI-VENEREAL WORK

In inquiring into this work I was greatly aided by M. Willen Schraener, the Secretary-General of *La Ligue Nationale Belge contre le Péril Vénérien.*

The measures adopted are somewhat similar to those in Great Britain, but differ in the much greater extent to which the services of private medical practitioners appear to be enrolled. The Belgian procedure is in the main the conception of Professor A. Bayet, the president of the league, on whose reports on the subject, as well as on my own inquiries, the following notes are based.

The expense of medicaments is borne entirely by the Government, that of the clinics by the provinces and communes, while social and propaganda work is a matter of private initiative. To the public clinics anyone can come for treatment. These clinics now number over 130.

The arseno-benzol preparations and certain bismuth and mercurial perparations, which are supplied to all approved physicians at the cost of the State, are dispensed by pharmacists, who are authorised to supply these to those doctors whose names are on a printed list distributed by the Commission Médicale Provinciale. In the nine provinces of

Belgium the last published list (January 1930) gives the names and addresses of 1,415 doctors, distributed as follows:—

Province of Antwerp	..	..	..	155
,, Brabant	..	..	..	366
,, West Flanders	..	..	..	142
,, East Flanders	..	..	..	142
,, Hainaut	..	..	..	242
,, Liège	..	..	..	202
,, Limbourg ..	..	..	..	66
,, Luxembourg	..	..	..	34
,, Namur	..	..	..	66

Thus about 27 per cent. of the practitioners in Belgium are entitled to receive gratuitous supply of approved arseno-benzol preparations.

Special stress is laid on this co-operation of private practitioners in the anti-venereal struggle, as forming an essential part of the programme. Professor Bayet emphasises the sterilisation of infection thus secured, and maintains that by this means the duration of infectivity of patients is reduced by four-fifths.

The work of pushing the work of the venereal disease clinics, of advising practitioners as to the possibility of obtaining arseno-benzol preparations for their poorly circumstanced patients, and of general propaganda is entrusted to the National League, which is actively engaged in this important work. Each year the league obtains returns from each clinic showing the number of patients treated. Although it is assumed that the treatment (including the drugs supplied to doctors) is intended for the poorer people, in practice treatment is given to all without social distinction.

The doctor treating private patients at the expense of the State is expected to accept possible supervision by a medical inspector of the Government, and is expected to make a return on which particulars of each case (not the name) are supplied. Doctors may not require the name of the patient coming to the clinic for treatment.

There is no complaint from practitioners of the operation

of these clinics, as the treatment of patients in private practice is recommended; and it would appear that this private treatment exceeds that given in the clinics.

Professor Bayet contrasts the utility of isolated clinics with that of private practitioners in combating venereal disease, to the partial disparagement of the former. He agrees that the specialised clinics at hospitals and dispensaries in great urban centres have a powerful influence; but even these "are too localised and are not effective for reducing syphilis wherever it prevails". Their range of action is too feeble. Even the smaller and more widely distributed dispensaries do not meet the need. Therapeutical sterilisation of the virus is the primary object and the chief means for overcoming syphilis, and for this purpose "the participation of the entire medical body is indispensable".

The statistics of Belgium show a great reduction in the incidence of syphilis. This runs on somewhat parallel lines to what has happened in Great Britain. It would appear, however, that in Belgium there has been no retardation in this decline in the last two years, such as is seen in the English statistics,[1] and perhaps one may justly state that in Great Britain dispensary treatment is more fully organised and more generally utilised than in Belgium, but that in the latter country there is more marked co-operation of private practitioners.

THE ORGANISATION OF THE MEDICAL PROFESSION

With few exceptions, doctors in Belgium are members of local or regional unions, known as *Syndicats médicaux* or *Collèges des Médecins*. These are federated into the Fédération Médicale Belge (National Union).

There is private medical practice, and, in addition, much contract work undertaken for mutualités. There are, furthermore, *Polycliniques* started and managed by groups of doctors, with a view to combined practice. At these the poor pay nothing, others a small fee.

Cliniques, or nursing-homes, are opened by individual

[1] But on this apparent retardation of decline in England, see Volume III.

doctors, or groups of doctors, or by religious orders, or the
Red Cross, or by philanthropists. In them acute medical and
particularly surgical cases requiring operation are treated.

These are private ventures, or are organised by associations.

In addition, there are the polycliniques [1] of the insurance
societies and the hospitals of the Committees for Public
Assistance appointed by the communal and provincial
authorities.

About one-half of the wage-earning people, industrial
and peasant, are members of mutualités, and these are
medically attended as described below. These mutualités
have initiated hospitals, dispensaries, and often sanatoria, in
supplementation of those provided by the State or local
authorities, or by the special organisations dealing with
child hygiene, tuberculosis, or venereal diseases.

Then there is in each commune medical assistance for the
destitute, the doctor being paid on the basis of a fee for
each consultation, or more often by an annual salary of a
few thousand francs. In Schaerbeck, for instance, with a
population of 112,000, four doctors are employed for
public assistance.

Nearly all medical services, except governmental posts,
are on a part-time basis.

The same doctor may be—

> Poor-law medical officer,
> Medical officer of health,
> School medical inspector,
> Medical officer of infant consultation, etc.

He may also be employed by the Accident Insurance Mutualité and by the Sickness Insurance Mutalités in his district.

Some employers of labour and some caisses communes,
as well as some municipalities, and some federations of
mutualités, employ whole-time doctors.

When institutional treatment is needed, this will be
obtained at the general hospital or hospitals provided in

[1] Polyclinics are dispensaries, including special departments for the separate
treatment of particular diseases. A polyvalent dispensary is a polyclinic.

each large community. In Brussels each of its nine boroughs has an independent municipal hospital, corresponding to its separate government. There appears to be no co-operation even for the treatment and isolation of infectious cases, but there is co-operation in the treatment of venereal diseases.

Many advanced cases of phthisis are treated in these municipal hospitals. Of the 200 beds at the Schaerbeck Hospital, some twenty-five to thirty were occupied by such cases.

At the general hospitals payment is exacted from each patient—3 francs for a consultation, and 35 francs per diem for in-patient maintenance. Some pay only a portion of this, the rest being paid by the commune. In Schaerbeck 25 per cent. of the patients pay the entire charge.

Two forms of insurance need to be differentiated, insurance for accident and for sickness.

ACCIDENT INSURANCE

For this the employer pays the entire premium, and the insurance may be special to a particular organisation, or secured from a general Accident Insurance Society. There is a strong opinion on the part of some doctors as well as of employers that accident insurance has prolonged the duration of incapacity for work after disablement. For instance, I was informed by one doctor that a broken leg, after which a man would formerly return to work in at least six weeks, now meant eight weeks' receipt of accident benefit. This does not necessarily imply that the recipient is a malingerer; but he is very apt to dramatise his injury, and to utilise less vigorously his will to get well. This tendency is exemplified in a recent notice—we might almost call it a warning notice—sent to its constituent medical confrères by the Federation of Medical Officers of Railways (F.M.O.). In this notice it is stated that the Société Nationale des Chemins de Fer (S.N.C.F.), to which the medical service is attached, has repeatedly drawn attention to the fact that since the new rule was introduced, giving free choice of doctors to the employees, the duration of absence from work after accident had considerably increased. This was attributed by the S.N.C.F. to the free choice of doctors and to the complaisance, which is the corollary of this free choice. The F.M.O. proceed to express their view that other factors than this are concerned; but, all the same, they urgently ask their confrères to return workers to work as soon as their condition permits this. They furthermore point out the importance of not damaging the cause of "free choice" by introducing argument as to certification, especially in view of the great difficulty the F.M.O. had experienced in securing this free choice.

SICKNESS INSURANCE

This is organised in large societies, which are independent, although subject to a few general conditions. They are subsidised by the Government. These societies are dominated by political or (and) religious considerations.

There are five chief National Unions of Sickness Insurance Societies, viz.:—

			Members [1]
Socialist National Union	..	.. ..	485,000
Catholic National Union	..	.. ..	337,000
Neutral National Union	..	.. ..	145,000
Employers' National Union..		.. ..	75,000
Liberal National Union	..	.. ..	65,000
			1,102,000

[1] Not including families.

Altogether there are 4,017 Approved Societies, of which —owing to consolidations—only 180 belong to the Socialist National Union. This union, although it comprises some 47 per cent. of the total insured, embraces these in 4½ per cent. of the Approved Societies.

Of the working classes about 50 per cent. are insured. To encourage sickness insurance the Government gives monetary grants. These include a minimum of 1·50 francs per month for each insured family for medical service.

Since 1922 this has been increased to 3 francs. The Government furthermore adds—

10 per cent. to the contributions for sickness benefit,
60 per cent. to the contributions for invalidity benefit.

It also doubles the fund for tuberculous work, and for maternity gives 50 francs for each birth, and adds 30 per cent. to the contribution of the mutualité for maternity, on condition that the mutualité pays at least 208 francs out of its funds. No distinction is made in respect of employed women.

The National Federation or Union of Socialists spent 113 million francs in 1928, 45 millions being paid by the Government for the five National Unions enumerated above.

Apparently there is no wage-limit for admission to a mutualité which receives official grants; but by the Bill for compulsory insurance now before the Belgian House of Representatives this is proposed to be limited to employed persons over 14 and under the age of 65, earning not more than 12,000 francs; the Socialists urging that it should apply to all those whose earnings are less than 24,000 francs per annum (about £137, or $685). The wage limit can be changed by Royal ordinance. Under this scheme administration will still be entrusted to approved insurance societies, the worker having free choice in joining these. The insured person will become eligible, not only for ordinary medical and surgical attendance, but also for recourse to specialist treatment. The various sickness and invalidity societies and their federations will be supervised by a Higher Council of twenty-seven members appointed by Royal decree, of which twelve will represent the insured, while medical and actuarial experts and representatives of the Government will also be included.

The contributions now paid vary according to the type of society. In one type a uniform payment is required, single men paying the same as married. This insures medical service for the wife and children, and maternity benefit for the wife. In a second type, a contribution is required on behalf of the wife and children as well as from the husband.

The sickness benefit may vary in the competitive societies from 6 to 25 francs per diem, according to the society to which the insured belongs. It continues for from three to six months. Similarly, invalidity insurance begins in the fourth or the seventh month of illness, according to the particular society of the insured person. Its amount varies from 4 to 12 francs a day. The method of paying weekly contributions varies. It may be collected at the insured person's home, or be received at a central office, or in industrial societies it may be deducted from the wages. The employer has no responsibility to affix the full amount of his employee's contribution in stamps to the official card, as in England. It must be noted that in Belgium employers do not contribute to sickness insurance, but they pay the entire cost of accident insurance. The benefit in accident insurance never exceeds 50 per cent. of the injured man's wages.

The *medical service* of each mutualité is separately organised, and varies in completeness.

Medical treatment includes the service of doctor and pharmacist, the insured person being expected to pay a fourth of the cost of medical treatment and of the cost of drugs. The amount of specialist and hospital service available varies in different societies.

Experience in recent years has shown considerable increase of sickness claims. M. Max Patteet, the secrétaire-adjoint of the Socialist National Union (L'Union Nationale des Fédérations de Mutualités Socialistes de Belgique), to whom and to Senator Jaunaiux, the general secretary of this union, I am indebted, thought that this increased demand for sickness benefit was a natural result of the propaganda and educational work of the union, insured persons seeking medical aid more readily than formerly.

Institutional treatment and treatment in polyclinics is usually organised by federations of mutualités. Thus the Socialist National Union has twenty-one federations, which take special charge of invalidity insurance.

At a polyclinic of the Socialist National Union in Brussels visited by me I found there were special physicians for respiratory diseases, for diseases of the nose, throat, and ears, for eye diseases, for surgery and gynæcological conditions.

The insured have the right to consult the part-time physicians of this clinic apart from any reference from their private doctor, an arrangement which can scarcely fail to induce undue recourse to the consultation centre, deficient co-operation with the private doctor, and redundant professional aid.

Special provision is made by mutualités for tuberculous patients. The Socialist National Union and the Union of Christian Democrats have colonies for feeble children. The National Catholic Union has a sanatorium of its own.

Remuneration of Insurance Doctors.—This is either on the plan of a fixed payment for each member for six months, at the end of which time the insured can change his doctor, or payment is made for medical work actually done. M. Patteet, looking at the problem from the standpoint of the federation, regarded the first method as failing to give the doctor an adequate inducement to do the best possible for his patient; while the second, which his federation preferred, was liable to lead to excessive medical attendance and certification. Each federation has a supervisory doctor. Some of these supervisors are whole-time officers of the mutualité. The free choice of doctor is gaining ground rapidly, and it appears certain that it will become general.

This free choice applies only to the general medical service. At the special clinics the doctors are appointed by the approved society. When hospital treatment is needed the approved society pays 50 per cent. of the cost of this, more or less, and the patient can choose his own hospital, which may be a private hospital, unless the approved society or federation has its own hospital service.

If the patient goes to a private hospital the surgeon who operates on him gives from 25 to 50 per cent. of his fee to the insurance doctor. The fees of the latter vary. They are from 7 to 12 francs for a consultation at the doctor's office, and 10 to 15 francs for each home visit (10 francs = about 13 pence, or 26 cents).

From what has been written it is clear that a large part of the total medical practice in Belgium is carried out for persons insured in sickness insurance societies. Including the families of the insured, who receive treatment under the conditions of insurance, the total thus treated must amount to half the entire population of Belgium.

A Bill is now under consideration by the Belgian legislature which will make sickness insurance generally compulsory. If that becomes law,. something like three-fourths of the total population will come within its provisions.

The views of the medical profession on present conditions of medical insurance practice are expressed through their national federation, and I have to thank Dr. Koettlitz, the secretary and president-elect of the Belgian Medical Federation, for valuable guidance in this matter.

The problem is wider than that of insurance. It affects also some branches of public health work. The Belgian medical profession do not like the extensions of public medical work. Recently there has been some effort to introduce specific immunisation against diphtheria, and there is a strong feeling that this work ought to be done by private practitioners. A protest against its being carried out by school doctors has recently been addressed to the municipalities by the National Union of Belgian Doctors. It is true that vaccination against smallpox is carried out by officials; but this is an established practice, the extension of which to other diseases is deprecated. Vaccination against smallpox is only indirectly compulsory. No child is admitted to school until he has been vaccinated.

I gathered that there was little or no objection to infant consultations, as the work in these is done by private practitioners. Furthermore, the medical fraternity have not the same distrust of a voluntary organisation as is entertained towards the Government or a municipality.

No objection is taken to the venereal disease clinics, for most patients prefer the private doctor, who in this respect is State-aided; and any doctor may secure admission to the official list.

Even so far as tuberculosis dispensaries are concerned, patients generally prefer their own doctor.

As regards treatment of insured persons, Dr. Koettlitz is confident that when compulsory insurance is introduced, nine-tenths of the medical profession will insist on payment based on actual work done, not implicating the doctor in the uncertainties of insurance. The contention is that insurance is for the patient and not for the doctor, and that the latter ought not to be involved in the risk.

To meet the increased certification experienced with free choice of doctor, it is agreed that the mutualité should exercise strong control by adequate supervision and checks.

The medical profession attach great importance not only to (1) free choice of doctor, and (2) to payment based on service rendered, the fee being paid directly to the doctor, but also (3) to the safeguarding of professional secrecy, and (4) the appointment as supervisors of medical practitioners chosen by insurance societies in consultation with the medical syndicates. They also contend that if disagreement arises this should be dealt with by committees on which the society and the medical syndicate should be equally represented.

As regards professional secrecy, it is agreed that exact medical certificates of cause of illness can be given by the attending physician to the medical supervisor of the mutualité.

The weekly contribution of employers is fixed under the Government's Bill at 2 per cent. of the worker's wage.

It will be seen that Belgium already has sickness insurance for the greater part of its wage-earning population, and that this insurance is on the point of being regularised and rendered compulsory for all employed persons below a certain wage. There is no intention in the impending legislation to abolish mutualités under private management, though it is strongly felt in many quarters that the present opportunity ought to be seized for this purpose. It is likely, however, that the large vested interests concerned will prevent this desirable object from being realised.

CHAPTER II

FRANCE[1]

PRELIMINARY SUMMARY

France is *par excellence* the country of centralised government, local initiative being hampered greatly. Voluntary social agencies are active in Paris, and to some extent elsewhere, in helping towards meeting the needs not officially supplied. Among recent official advances the most noteworthy is the provision for social hygiene dispensaries[2] at which patients with tuberculosis, venereal disease, suspected cancer, as well as mothers and their infants, are advised and to some extent treated.

The French medical profession holds rigid views as to medical secrecy, and the new law for sickness insurance presents great initial difficulties. For similar reasons anti-tuberculosis work is seriously hampered. Notwithstanding strenuous effort by special grants to promote maternal health and favour larger families, there is serious deficiency of child welfare work and of work in the hygiene of school children. The details in regard to hospital treatment and the care of the sick poor scarcely lend themselves to summary. General and local details are given in the following pages.

France, a leader in some of the arts of civilisation, presents strange defects and anomalies in its medico-hygienic administration. It is not surprising that Calmette, quoted by Drs. Spillman and Parisot, has asked why, and by what strange aberration, the country of Pasteur has not been the first to profit by the beneficent results of his work. Calmette continued: Why should it be that social hygiene is less advanced in France than abroad, and that a comparison of what has been done in France and in other countries is disadvantageous to France?

[1] Date of investigation, March 1929.
[2] The term "Social Hygiene" in this volume is not used in the more restricted sense of the work done by the American and English Association of Social Hygiene. The French and other European Social Hygienic Dispensaries concern themselves with maternity and child welfare, with tuberculosis, venereal disease, cancer, and often with alcoholism.

And yet, in some respects, other countries may learn much from the progress of events bearing on the prevention and treatment of disease in France.

Before the salient features of these events—so far as they bear on the relation between clinical and preventive medicine, between private and public medicine—can be understood in their setting, it is needful to understand something of government in France. Although this is a tangled and complicated combination of centralisation with a minimum of local autonomy, and of official agencies with related or independent voluntary organisations, a sketch of these diverse conditions must be attempted.

CENTRAL AND LOCAL GOVERNMENT

There are three administrative degrees: the general administration of the State, that of the département, and that of the commune. Universal male suffrage gives some control of the electorate over central administration and perhaps less control (chiefly in the direction of limiting or increasing the budget) over local administration.

The Central Government, in the decisions of its own Cabinet (Committee of Ministers), is guided in part by the Council of State (Conseil d'Etat), which helps in considering and elucidating legislative and administrative problems as they arise. It is composed of legal and administrative experts.

In technical matters the Ministry is assisted by le Conseil supérieur d'Hygiène de France.

Similarly there is a Conseil supérieur de l'Assistance Publique, as well as a Conseil supérieur de la Natalité, Conseil supérieur de la Protection de l'Enfance, Commission supérieure de la Tuberculose, etc.

The most important of these is the Conseil supérieur de l'Hygiène, which comprises members nominated by the Minister who represents the State and twenty-five members nominated from doctors, lawyers, engineers, chemists, etc.

It is the duty of this council to investigate questions referred to it and those on which, e.g. epidemics, its advice is obligatory. It is doubtful if such a "standing" council is so advantageous in the public interest as would be committees appointed to consider each special problem as it arises and especially competent in respect of that problem. Furthermore, dependence for expert assistance on such a council suggests with much probability the need for a permanent technical staff in each Department of the Government competent to give in most respects the needed guidance. The need for such a skilled staff on an adequate scale appears to be one of the most urgent needs of French administration.

Locally, France is divided into 90 continental départements, which are subdivided into about 3,000 cantons, and these again into nearly 27,000 communes. The département is headed by the prefect (préfet), who is nominated by the Minister of the Interior and appointed by the President, and is really the political representative of the Government. He is the sole responsible executive and is appointed without time limit. He appoints all subordinate officials, including school teachers, and has wide police and public health powers, including large control over the communes and their mayors.

Associated with the préfet is the Conseil de Préfecture, consisting of three members appointed by the Central Government. They have a small salary, are usually lawyers, and they advise the préfet, who need not adopt their advice. They deputise for him.

There is also a Départemental Conseil-Général consisting of from 17 to 67 members, each canton sending one member. These are appointed for six years, half of them retiring every three years. They elect their own chairman. Their functions are defined by the Central Parliament (la Chambre des Députés and Le Sénat), and include the assessing of the taxes for each arrondissement, the fixing of departmental taxes, roads, training colleges for teachers, and the provision for the destitute and for children and for lunacy.

The population of départements varies from 89,000 to 4½ millions.

The departmental unit of local government is the commune; each commune, whether a village or a borough, being
on an equal footing. Some 22,000 of these in the year 1921
had a population of 500 or less.

The commune has a Conseil municipal, consisting of
10 to 36 members according to population, elected for
four years by universal male adult suffrage. It has restricted
powers of government and taxation, subject to the approval
of the préfet, who can suspend it, while the Central Government can dissolve it. The communal mayor is elected for
four years by the ballot of the council. He is unpaid, and
very commonly is re-elected. The mayor's secretary is
usually the local schoolmaster.

The canton and the arrondissement stand between the
département and the commune. The canton is a group of
communes for certain judicial purposes and for elections.
The arrondissement is an administrative subdivision of
the département.

The general system is one of bureaucratic centralisation
for the whole country, the préfet being the chief person to
ensure this. Historically, its object was to unify the
government of the entire country; in the present stage
it implies a shackling of local enterprise, and an influence
tending to keep at a very low ebb the training of local
patriotism.[1]

The French system is important, among other reasons
because in Belgium, Holland, and Italy closely resembling
systems prevail. In Scandinavian countries also the French
model has been partly followed.

[1] The following extract from Professor Joseph Barthélemy's *Le Gouverne-
ment de la France* (Payot, Paris, 1924) illustrates the general statement
made above:—
    "The municipal council cannot, without the approbation of the préfet,
change the name of a street! . . . If a public lavatory is needed, this may
involve an addition to the budget and the central power must approve.
. . . On the other hand, there is compulsory local expenditure. . . . For
several years the Municipal Council of Paris refused the police budget,
which was enforced, but they lost any control over the police."
    After pleading for decentralisation as a school of public life, M. J.
Barthélemy strikes a warning note as to excessive local liberty . . . "when
one is cold, warmth is desirable, but one need not throw oneself in the
fire".

The arrangements may be made clearer by the following scheme:—

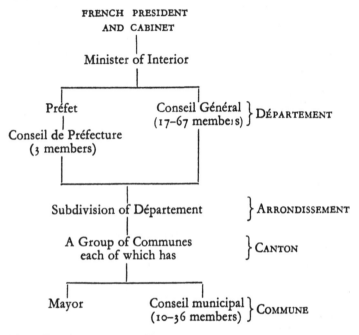

THE GOVERNMENT OF PARIS

Paris has an organisation which may be roughly summarised as follows: It is combined for some purposes with that of the Département of the Seine. The population of Paris proper at the census of 1926 was 2,838,416; that of the entire département was 4,567,690. The Préfet of the Seine is Mayor of Paris, except for police purposes, and also exercises the usual functions of a préfet in the entire département. The Préfet of Police is a colleague and not a subordinate of the Préfet of the Seine.

The Municipal Council of Paris has eighty members. These are elected by manhood suffrage for four years and are paid. They are subdivided into six standing committees, with occasional special committees. Their functions are almost solely advisory, and they are in nearly all respects subordinate to the will of the two préfets. Paris is subdivided into twenty arrondissements, each having its own mayor.

The Département of the Seine has a Conseil Général consisting of the eighty members of the Conseil municipal, together with forty members from the two arrondissements outside Paris. Government approval is required for most of its decisions.

Advisory Boards are largely used for the whole of Paris and for each of its twenty arrondissements. These meet regularly, and are consulted on various branches of public health. They include representatives of the Central Government and of the municipality, as well as ex-officio members, representing various expert divisions of work.

PUBLIC ASSISTANCE

Public Assistance, including the administration of hospitals, asylums, etc., is supervised by a board consisting of the two préfets and eighteen others, of whom eleven have certain qualifications, while five are appointed by the President of the Republic and two are members of the municipal council. In each arrondissement there is a Bureau de Bienfaisance, consisting of the mayor of the arrondissement and of twelve others. Each arrondissement again is divided into twelve districts, each of which is under one member of the Bureau de Bienfaisance.

The work of the Public Assistance forms a very large part of the medico-hygienic service of the State. Its magnitude for Paris may be gathered from the following illustrative facts and figures, taken from the *Compte Moral et Administratif de l'Exercise*, 1926 (Administration Générale de l'Assistance Publique á Paris). This is the most recent report available. The service has existed since 1803.

YEAR 1926

No. of days of patients in hospitals	6,601,000
No. of patients admitted after examination in hospital consultations	194,000
Total number of consultations	2,906,000
General and special cost of hospitals (French francs)	222,015,000
Repayment of cost of patients in hospitals and retreats (French francs)	31,434,000

The municipal hospitals suffer from overcrowding, especially during the winter, and the nursing service is not yet completely developed. In January 1927 there were 3,955 medical and 3,078 surgical beds.

Puericulture.—In 1926, 14,738 infants attended institutions of puericulture, the number of consultations being 65,215. These institutions are being increasingly used in the training of medical students, of nurses, and for instructing girls in communal schools.

Maternity.—Of 61,500 confinements in Paris in 1926,

40,387 were in charge of the Assistance Publique, or 65·7 per cent., viz.,
27,142 in hospitals,
10,010 by approved midwives,
3,235 by midwives of Bureaux de Bienfaisance.

On their leaving maternity homes, and as allocations, the amount given to mothers in 1926 was 1,903,706 francs. The succour given to mothers for their infant children totalled 4,395,107 francs.

The number of confinements in hospitals has increased in recent years; the number attended by midwives is almost stationary.

The anti-tuberculosis and anti-venereal organisations of the Public Assistance will be described later.

The aid given in parturition is generous, and since 1917 restrictions to succour to women in their confinements based on family income have fallen almost into desuetude in Paris.

PROTECTION DE LA MATERNITÉ

The French law for the Protection de la Maternité may be summarised at this point. It has important bearings on the relation of the medical profession to the public health.

An enactment of July 15, 1893, included lying-in women amongst those having the right to gratuitous medical aid from the A.P.,[1] their condition being placed in the same category as disabling sickness. This assistance, the law

[1] L'Assistance Publique.

specified, may be given at home, or if "useful" care cannot be given at home, then in a hospital. The care includes a doctor, medicines, and appliances. The law of June 17, 1913 (Strauss law), made rest during the month after parturition obligatory for women gainfully employed. By the first article of this enactment, women evidently pregnant can leave their employer without giving notice, and without any obligation to pay an indemnity in lieu of leave.

Then follows for all industrial and commercial occupations, also for professional and charitable posts, the following: "It is forbidden to employ women during the four weeks following childbirth."

Article 3 of Strauss law provides for a daily monetary allowance during the period of rest from salaried work preceding and following childbirth. Before childbirth a medical certificate is required to the effect that she cannot continue work without danger to herself and her infant. Application at the bureau of A.P. with the necessary certificate is required to obtain this benefit. The benefit was extended in 1919 to every woman, salaried or not, provided that she is without adequate resources; and a further enactment dated January 1928 has fixed the total duration of rest before and after confinement at twelve weeks. The benefit very appropriately is subject to required conditions as to rest and hygiene. This opens up important future opportunities for maternal and infant care.

The municipal council decides for each commune the allowance to be made, subject to approval of the préfet. The scale before the war varied from 0.50 to 1.50 francs a day. If more than 1.50 francs, the excess was to be paid at the exclusive cost of the commune. The French budget for 1930 fixes the daily grant at 1.50 francs. In 1927, 304,487 mothers obtained the benefit under the Strauss law.

In 1913 the above service was made obligatory on the départements, in association with the communes and the State. The potential value of the service has been made real in large measure by the antenatal consultations attached to the maternity hospitals of the A.P., and by official maisons maternelles and cantines maternelles, and by various voluntary agencies.

Two forms of assistance have been provided by legislation after the infant's birth, in addition to the small monetary allowance named above.

The law of October 24, 1919, initiated

primes d'allaitement

bonuses for continued maternal lactation of 15 francs, payable each month during the twelve months following childbirth. In 1927 the number of mothers receiving primes d'allaitement was 267,484. Under the new law of Social Insurance, primes d'allaitement will begin at 100 francs and gradually decrease to 15 francs a month at the end of the year. These bonuses are only given to women already in receipt of the benefits provided for women at their confinement. Dames visiteuses are sometimes provided to supervise the administration of this work. Otherwise a medical certificate of continuation of lactation is required.

On August 5, 1917, a law was passed to facilitate breast-feeding in places of work. This law made it obligatory in establishments employing more than one hundred women aged over fifteen years to provide accommodation and allow two intervals of thirty minutes each during which mothers could suckle their infants. Relatively small use has been made of this law.

Encouragement à la Natalité

has also been the subject of much further legislation, in addition to the enactments already enumerated. In the cost of these measures the State shares with the département and the communes.

1. By the law of April 30, 1920, two additional bonuses are forthcoming: (a) one of 100 francs or more at the birth of each child beyond the second; (b) a second bonus, which is a form of insurance, the amount given not being less than 500 or more than 1,000 francs, one-half being devoted to regular payments to the parents, and the other being an insurance for the contingency of parental death

or accruing to the child when he becomes 25 years old. These forms of assistance are held not to constitute charity. They can be claimed for all children. The amount given for successive children varies in different municipalities. The State gives a subvention in aid of these grants.

2. By the law of July 20, 1923, further encouragement of complete families has been accorded. It enacts that in families of more than three children an annual grant shall be given for each child beyond the third who is less than 13 years old. The amount is fixed at 360 francs a year for each of such children. This is independent of other grants.

3. Under an Act of March 22, 1924, a deduction of 3,000 francs from family income is allowed for children before tax is imposed on the basis of income. Other deductions of an allied kind are made.

In the budget for 1930, 42 million francs are reserved for assistance to women in childbirth, 63·2 million francs for primes d'allaitement, 11 millions for subventions to organisations for maternity and child welfare, and 3 millions for the needs of the Roussel law. (Information supplied by the Office National d'Hygiène Publique, based on the report of M. Landry to the Budget Commission of the Chambre des Députés.)

VOLUNTARY ORGANISATIONS

Private charity takes a large—and commonly a preponderant—part in France in regard to help in childbirth, as well as in puericulture, and in measures for the prevention and treatment of tuberculosis and venereal diseases. There are too many private societies giving varied help, and it is fairly clear that economy of effort and of money would be secured by large amalgamations of these societies. The policy of official France has always been to encourage voluntary help, and evidently the need for voluntary effort must continue in view of the parsimony in official help, especially in help other than for maternity. Outside Paris and a few other cities the ineffectiveness and inadequacy of official hospital and dispensary provision are particularly evident. Given adequacy as well as full efficiency of effort, official and voluntary, the combination can be excellent. M. Landry's statement on this point may be quoted:—

For certain tasks, private organisations are superior to public official activities in the suppleness which enables them to adapt themselves more easily to circumstances. Those directing these private organisations work in a disinterested manner, and are animated by a zeal which is not always seen to the same degree in administrative work.

Disinterested action ought to be practicable in official work; nor need there be less zeal in such work than in that of voluntary organisations.

It is impossible to describe many of the voluntary organisations here; but some having national importance are mentioned at this point, as they are in intimate and invaluable relation with official agencies.

First may be mentioned—

L'Office National d'Hygiène Sociale (O.N.H.S.).—This owes its foundation and present financial position to the Rockefeller Foundation, which contributes annually a share of the cost of maintenance of L'Office.

By a ministerial decree dated December 4, 1924, the creation of the office was authorised, and it has become a quasi-governmental department, reporting annually as to its work to the Ministry of Labour and Health.

It fulfils the following functions:—

1. It collects, summarises, and makes readily available documentation of all available information on hygiene and social medical activities in France: of the dossiers made available to visitors I wish here to express my high appreciation.

2. It acts as a central educational agent, helping the educational efforts of various health organisations in France and its colonies.

3. It helps in various ways in ensuring a liaison between private and public organisations, in the interest of the public health.

Associations d'Hygiène Sociale are to be found throughout France, of which that for the Département de L'Aisne may be taken as an example. It is the direct successor[1] of the American Committee for the devastated regions of France, and owes much, as does public health work generally in the département, to the work of that committee. The préfet, in addressing the last Annual Meeting of the above A.H.S., laid stress on the fact that the basis of its organisation was "to respect, above all, private endeavours", and this view is evident throughout France. The aims of the A.H.S. are to develop already existent hygienic-social measures, and to extend the field of action of the infirmière-visiteuse (health visitor or public health nurse). In pursuing these aims the A.H.S. for the Aisne helps in the work of prenatal and puerperal hygiene and the hygiene of the infant, and in work for the pre-school child and the scholar. In the Annual Report of the A.H.S. it is difficult to distinguish between its activities and those of the officials of the département in public health work; but the nurses are provided largely by the A.H.S.; and their work, especially as regards means of locomotion, continues to be subsidised by the Rockefeller Foundation. (For further particulars, see the account of my visit to Soissons and Laon, page 104).

The headquarters of the *League of Red Cross Societies* are in Paris, and to the secretary-general (M. T. B. Kittredge) and his colleagues I am indebted for help in securing touch with various public health organisations. Dr. F. Humbert, director of the health division, League of Red Cross Societies, accompanied me on various visits, and to his guidance I owe much.

Between the O.N.H.S. and various other voluntary organisations a close liaison exists. I can only enumerate some of them:—

Le Comité National de l'Enfance,
Le Comité National de Défense contre la Tuberculose,
Le Comité National des Œuvres de plein air,
La Ligue National contre le Péril Vénérien,
La Ligue National contre l'Alcoolisme,
La Ligue d'Hygiène mentale,
Les Camps de Vacances, etc.

[1] Described as "la fille et le successeur" in the Report of the A.H.S.

I may now describe briefly the combined official and voluntary medical services, in connection with which friction between private and medical practitioners may arise. These services relate chiefly to the care of maternity and of infants, the inspection and treatment of scholars, and the diagnosis and treatment of tuberculosis and venereal diseases. There will be added shortly medical sickness insurance, on which reference, should be made to page 90 and to my discussion of "Le Secret Médical" (page 96).

MATERNITY MEDICAL CARE.

The vast extent of gratuitous medical aid for maternity in Paris has already been indicated; and throughout France this form of medical aid is given with generosity by public authorities, either at home or in maternity hospitals, or in detached divisions of general municipal hospitals.

In the Paris hospitals belonging to the Assistance Publique the maternity provision is usually admirable.

Most patients are treated gratuitously, but women with means are expected to pay. Nearly 66 per cent. of births in Paris occur in the service of the Assistance Publique, either in hospital or through the midwives of the hospitals or municipality (page 50).

Antenatal consultations are always gratuitous in Paris, and private doctors do not appear to object to this, as they sometimes do in the provinces.

I visited the Clinic Baudelocque, accompanied by Dr. Humbert, and was received by Professor Couvelaire, the head of the clinic. This clinic has 200 beds and 70 cots, and is admirably arranged. There is an Infant Consultation attached to it. Extract from *Annual Report*:—

Number of confinements at this clinic 2,431
Number of consultations antenatally 13,326
Number of women consulting antenatally 5,492
Number of women referred to the Dispensary for
    Syphilitics 399
Number of women tuberculous or suspects referred to
    T.B. Dispensary 142

This clinic contains two important special divisions. In one, syphilitic lying-in or expectant mothers are treated, and in the other special provision is made for consumptives, who are confined in a separate pavilion. This work was begun in 1921, and arrangements have been made for the separation of the infant from the mother, with the latter's consent, and its placing out in a healthy home. The work of immediate separation of infants from their tuberculous mothers was initiated by Professor Léon Bernard, Professor of Phthisiology at the Hospital Laennec, who also initiated L'Œuvre du Placement Familiale des Tout-Petits.

Professor Couvelaire (in *Gynécologie et Obstetrique*, t. xiii, No. 6, juin 1926) gives the following figures of arrangements made by L'Œuvre du Placement Familiale des Tout-Petits for such newborn infants of tuberculous parents in the year 1926:—

From the Clinique Baudelocque ..	50 infants
From other Maternity Hospitals in Paris	9 infants

The Baudelocque clinic receives voluntary social assistance from two organisations. The first of these is special to the clinic, and arranges for help for the poor, for the distribution of layettes, and for the reception of selected children of the poor, aged 1 to 3 years, after weaning, preference being given to cases of congenital syphilis. The second society is the Service social à l'Hôpital, which inquires into the material and social conditions of each applicant to the hospital from a medical as well as a social point of view.

Sage-Femmes.—Midwives and untrained women, "handy women", attend the majority of births in France. Their distribution may be gathered from the following examples taken from official statistics. There are from 11,000 to 12,000 midwives in France, or about 1 to 3,285 of population. The low birth-rate of France must be borne in mind. The proportion varies greatly in different départements.

Thus, in—

				Proportion to Population
Seine ..	..	..	..	.. 1 to 4,119
Seine-Inférieure	..	..	..	1 to 7,316
Seine-et-Marne	..	..	..	1 to 6,126
Seine-et-Oise	..	..	..	1 to 5,946

The fewest number of midwives are in the départements of

				Proportion to Population
Orne ..	..	..	..	.. 1 to 13,740
Manche	..	..	..	1 to 12,515
Côtes-du-Nord	..	..	..	1 to 15,495
Corsica	..	..	..	1 to 14,744

and the largest proportions of midwives are in—

				Proportion to Population
Rhin (bas)	..	..	..	.. 1 to 1,178
Rhin (haut)	..	..	..	1 to 1,317
Gironde	..	..	..	1 to 1,127

The law of November 30, 1892, forbids the practice of midwifery except by those having diplomas furnished by the Government of France as the result of an examination before a faculty of medicine or a school recognised for this purpose. This law appears not to be always enforced, especially in rural areas. The diploma is given after two yearly examinations. By a decree of January 9, 1917, the diploma can only be obtained after two years' study, the second year being spent in a maternity institution authorised for this purpose.

Article 4 of the same enactment forbids the midwife to use instruments, and makes it her duty, in difficult labour, to send for a doctor or health officer. No special provision is made for paying the doctor thus sent for, except under the general law for gratuitous medical attendance (page 61), which appears to involve the necessity for prevision and prearrangement if a doctor is to be ensured. It also implies the existence of destitution. Professor Couvelaire informed me that in Paris such complicated cases were all admitted to his clinic or to one of the many other maternity hospitals in Paris. This appears to be regarded as meeting the needs of the case; but, if English experience is a guide, it appears probable that behind this difficulty in obtaining domiciliary medical help in parturition there must be much avoidable suffering, or at least suffering that could be greatly reduced.

Professor Couvelaire informed me, and I received the same information in other parts of France, that, with diminishing indigence in the population, doctors are being employed in an increasing number of confinements. This appears to arise from the view that it is more *chic* to employ a doctor than a midwife.

Midwives are not allowed to give drugs; but an exception is made as to a silver solution for the eyes of newborn infants.

I do not give any statistics here as to puerperal mortality, as it is doubtful whether throughout France the records give a correct representation of the true position.

There is no doubt as to the essential facts. Parturition in civilised communities is associated in a considerable proportion of the total births with danger to life or to physical health. This danger can be avoided in a large proportion of cases, given prescient and adequate skilled guidance. In France commonly this is not given, and the continuance in practice of "handy women" is tolerated, while the law to prevent this already exists. To enforce the law against such unqualified practice would necessitate large expenditure by the communes on obstetric aid for those who are destitute in this specific sense; and that aid commonly is not forthcoming, or is only available under the humiliating condition of anticipatory application to the mayor's office for the necessary authorisation.

An adequate subsidised service of qualified midwives throughout France would constitute an immense sanitary reform. In view of the other generous provisions made by France in aid of maternity, it is surprising that this is not given; and especially it is surprising that the availability of skilled medical aid in obstetric complications continues to be hemmed in by difficulties in the way of previous official authorisation. How far these instructions are waived in unexpected emergencies is open to doubt.

A report by Mlle Mossé, Sage-femme-en-chef de la Maternité de Paris (April 5, 1926), for a copy of which I am indebted to the Research Division of L'Office National d'Hygiène Sociale, may be quoted as throwing valuable light on the potential value of an adequate midwifery service, especially in rural districts. While in the great towns the supply of midwives is excessive, in small communities they cannot unaided "make a living"; and the recommendation made by Mlle Mossé, that midwives in rural districts should be made also the agents of social hygiene as health visitors (infirmières-visiteuses), is one which has been adopted in some parts of rural England. A relatively small addition to the training of midwives would render this practicable. In England midwife visitors are also usually qualified as nurses.

The combination in one person of the functions of midwife and of public health nurse or health visitor appears to offer the best prospect of a rapid improvement in puericulture in rural France.

So many forms of medico-hygienic work, including the protection of maternity and infancy, are closely related to the activities of

L'ASSISTANCE PUBLIQUE

as to make further notes (see page 49) on it desirable, before describing further efforts for child welfare and anti-tuberculosis and anti-syphilis work.

The hospitals in France, outside the great cities, are not satisfactory institutions, and even in those cities they are often overcrowded and inadequate. Skilled nursing is not always provided. Some of the hospital clinics in Paris are models of what should be provided both structurally and functionally.

Hospitals are provided in communes by the municipality, and the sick of that commune needing hospital treatment have an implied right to admission. Whether payment shall be demanded depends on the social circumstances of the patient.

In towns there may be considerable relaxation of the rules as to admission to hospitals of those not inscribed on the list of the A.M.G. (Assistance Médicale Gratuité). In Paris there is no restriction on the admission of pregnant or parturient women.

In 1919, in 87 départements, there were 1,260 hospitals possessing 178,355 beds.

Regulations for Free Medical Attendance.—1. *Saône-et-Loire.* —So far as free domiciliary medical attendance and hospital treatment are concerned, the regulations of the Service d'Assistance Médicale Gratuité of the Département of Saône-et-Loire may be outlined in illustration. This département ment only two years ago agreed to the principle of "free choice of doctors" for the destitute, being almost the last of the départements of France to adopt this, which is now the general rule. The rules for regulating this service provide for the giving gratuitously at the patient's home, for patients "privé de ressources", of medical, surgical, pharmaceutical, and obstetric aid; and for giving similar services in a hospital when the patient cannot be properly treated at home.

Three categories of persons to be assisted are recognised:—

(*a*) Totally indigent, to whom complete aid is given;

(*b*) Semi-indigent, who, in a protracted illness are given medical services at home or in hospital, but are expected to pay for drugs, etc.; and

(*c*) Persons who are entitled to hospital treatment, because they cannot afford the expense of treatment which is protracted, and which necessitates admission to a hospital.

A list of doctors, chemists, and midwives who have accepted the tariffs and other conditions of the official service is published each year. The person assisted can make his choice from this list, limited by the requirement that the one geographically most convenient should be chosen. The professional service is subject to conditions imposed by the préfet, on the advice of a Commission of Control.

A list of persons who in case of illness are entitled to medical assistance is sent by the Administrative Commission of the Bureau of Assistance to the municipal council, and is revised quarterly. Doctors are expected to help in making up this list. If they cannot attend the conference at which the list is prepared, they are expected to give the mayor a list of those persons recommended by them for gratuitous treatment. In addition—and this has special interest as bearing on an attempt to secure co-operation with the organisations of private medicine—the Departmental Federation, or syndicate of doctors, is expected to send observations on the medical assistance given.

Those desiring to be inscribed on the list of eligibles for gratuitous treatment are expected to supply full information as to family income. The doctor chosen by the indigent must be the nearest available physician; but all the doctors in a single town, borough, or village (*ville, bourg, village*) are deemed equally near.

In defining indigence, it is specified that infants and young children need not appear on the official list, "for sickness of the child does not deprive the family of resources"—a statement on the latent potentialities for evil of which one need not animadvert.

The list of possible recipients of medical relief is debated by the municipal council in secret committee. This list, when approved, is deposited in the mayor's office and with the doctors concerned. A place on the list holds good for a year.

As regards *domiciliary* help, a patient cannot change his doctor during a given illness without the consent of this doctor and the authorisation of the Bureau of Assistance. The doctor keeps dossiers of three different colours, according to the class of patient. Visits are made only if the patient cannot attend the doctor's cabinet.

For *hospital* help the hospital available is decided on general lines by a general council for several communes.

A patient can only be admitted on a certificate signed by the doctor and countersigned by the mayor, indicating that he is on the list of those eligible for assistance, and stating the nature of his illness. Unless it is adequately relaxed in emergencies, this condition evidently may be mischievous.

A tariff of medical fees is given in the regulations from which the preceding brief extracts have been made. For home consultations the medical fee is 6 francs; for home visits in the day 8 francs,[1] at night 16 francs, with extra allowance for excessive distances. The tariff for various operations is also on a low scale.

2. *Hérault.*—In the Département of Hérault somewhat similar regulations exist. The present regulations were made in 1923.

The service is entrusted to all the doctors in the département who accept its conditions. Each person assisted can choose his own doctor, but only doctors and midwives who are nearest the patient's home are obliged to respond to calls. At the consultations held in the departmental dispensary, the patient can consult any doctor serving there.

The patient must not be sent to a hospital "unless it is absolutely impossible to treat him at home"; and the order for admission, signed by the doctor and the chief of the Assistance Bureau, ought to give the reasons for this impossibility.

When a patient wishes to consult a doctor at the latter's residence, he receives a card from the mayor (*bon de consultation*).

A card is required from the mayor for attendance in accouchement.

Similarly for home visits of a doctor, a representative of the patient indicates the name of the doctor desired, and receives a *feuille de maladie*, on which the doctor is required to enter his visits and prescriptions. The doctor need not visit the patient again, unless his previous visit has been

[1] 125 francs = one pound sterling, or about $4.7.

viséd by the mayor. This is done after each visit by the representative of the patient.

The regulations as to economy of prescriptions need not be detailed, nor the regulations for pharmacists.

For each visit 5 francs, and for each consultation 4 francs, are paid, with an added allowance of 2 francs per kilometre for travelling, not including return.[1]

Midwives are paid 20 francs a case when delivery is in the midwife's house, and 30 francs elsewhere. This fee includes three visits during the eight days after confinement.

If there is no midwife within 12 kilometres a doctor can be called in, who receives 120 francs for attendance.[1]

Accounts for payment are required to be presented three times a year.

It appears clear that the system briefly outlined in the two instances given above encourages restricted utilisation of medical aid either at home or in hospitals. Emergency provisions exist; but the service is not likely to be popular or to meet public needs under the official safeguarding, the signing and countersigning of documents, and the possible purging of the list of recommended cases which the regulations involve.

The way is now clear for an outline of some other special medical measures in which voluntary and official agencies co-operate. These relate especially to Infant Welfare Work, and to Consultations for Tuberculosis and Venereal Diseases. The official work of school and medical inspection will then be noted.

INFANT WELFARE WORK

Much of this work is official, as already indicated, and is controlled centrally by the Minister of Health, of Assistance, and of Social Insurance, under one or other of the two divisions of Administration of Assistance or Public Health.

---

[1] In 1928 the medical fee for a visit or a consultation was increased to 8 francs, and for accouchements 120 francs.

The following Voluntary Societies take an active part in this work:—

The *League against Infant Mortality* has associated with it the honoured names of Roussel, Budin, and Strauss; and in extending its work there has recently been formed the *National Infancy Committee*.

Consultations de Nourissons are numerous, and closely related to these are *Gouttes de Lait*. In my visit to Laon, in the Département of Aisne, I found an excellent institution having the double title, the consultations being a special division of the work, which included also the supply of bottled milk. It was emphasised that this was done in a manner which would not favour recourse to artificial feeding. No special treatment is given, but hygienic advice and propaganda.

Vaccination against Tuberculosis forms an exception to the rule of no treatment at infant consultations. This vaccination is not limited to infants attending the consultation.

In most parts of France the mothers still bring chiefly sick infants to the consultations. Nine thousand addresses are published in *Paris Bienfaisant, Charitable et Sociale* of agencies for promoting Infant Welfare; nevertheless they are inadequate and inco-ordinated. *Pouponnières* (residential crèches) of the Département of Seine have some 300 beds, while each year 9,000 to 10,000 infants are placed out to nurse. 117 crèches et chambres d'allaitement of this départe- ment had 3,879 places for children under three years in 1923 (figures given by Mlle Dr. Labeaume). Results could be much improved if all organisations were federated. Attempts at co-operation have been only partially successful; and the same remark, it may be added, applies to anti- tuberculosis work.

Prenatal Consultations

At the Goutte de Lait at Soissons (Saône) visited by me, *Prenatal Consultations* also are held. Last year they numbered sixty-three. Few cases are sent by private physicians; many patients are received at these and at postnatal consultations because certification is required for paying nursing mothers for abstaining from work and for bonuses for continued lactation. Sometimes attendance at the consultation is made a condition of receipt of these benefits.

In the whole of the Département of the Aisne eight to ten thousand births occur annually, and some three thousand infants and their mothers attend infant consultations. Each commune can receive help from départemental funds for the establishment of a consultation, given a minimum standard of attendance. Throughout the département private medical practitioners conduct these consultations and are paid for their services. If several doctors live in the same commune a rotation of not less than a year is sometimes allowed; usually it can be arranged for one doctor to act indefinitely.

At Soissons, as seen above, prenatal consultations are arranged at the Goutte de Lait. In the rest of the Département of the Aisne, Dr. Chapuis, the Director of the Public Health Services in the département, has arranged for such consultations to be given in the private office of any doctor chosen by the expectant mother herself. The arrangement is ingenious and should do much good. Its possibilities for good are, however, limited by the fact that the recipient of this help must have previously applied at the mairie and been inscribed on the list of the Bureau de Bienfaisance for gratuitous medical help. Women whose husbands do not pay income tax can have this boon, which implies that three-fourths of the total population are eligible for it. The département pays 10 francs each for three medical examinations during each pregnancy. The document in which recourse to this help is advised is given on the opposite page in an English dress. So far only a limited recourse has been had to these consultations.

In the départemental studies some further particulars of public medical care of infants and children are given. The amount of work done at the public expense (official and voluntary) varies greatly in different parts of France.

One cannot fail to be struck by the amount of care

DÉPARTEMENT DE L'AISNE

DIRECTION DÉPARTEMENTALE D'HYGIÈNE
MEDICAL SUPERVISION DURING PREGNANCY

Expectant Mothers!

In a woman pregnancy is a condition which should call forth all her care.

Many pathological incidents manifest themselves or start during pregnancy, and may have disastrous effects on the health of the expectant mother or of the future child.

Medical supervision during pregnancy is the only means of recognising in time complications which may have to be dealt with, and of ensuring early enough the treatment necessary to ensure the health of the mother and the unborn child.

The Conseil Général de l'Aisne, the Ministère de l'Hygiène, and l'Office d'Hygiène sociale de l'Aisne have joined forces with the medical profession in the département to provide a service of gratuitous consultations for medical supervision during pregnancy, to be carried out as follows:—

Working of the Service

Pregnant women, whose names have been entered at the Assistance Médicale Gratuite or at a Bureau de Bienfaisance which has funds for this purpose, should present themselves at the mairie of their commune, where they will be given a maternity voucher.

Pregnant women belonging to a family of which the head does not pay taxes, and who wish to benefit by these consultations, must first obtain a certificate that they are exempt from taxation. This certificate should be asked for from the collector of taxes of the commune, who will give it gratuitously. This certificate they can exchange at the mairie for a maternity voucher. This voucher entitles them, after the third month of pregnancy, to three free consultations—one during the third month, one during the fifth month, and the last during the eighth month of pregnancy—with free choice of doctor. All further information is given in the maternity voucher.

To avoid publicity it is not obligatory for unmarried mothers to go to the mairie to procure a maternity voucher. They may go straight to the doctor of their own choice, who will himself give them the maternity voucher.

In your own interests, in that of our Race,

Make Use of These Consultations

bestowed by charitable and official agencies upon neglected and deserted children, and the comparative paucity of this extra-familial care for the children in normal family life, for whom the greatest national good could be achieved. This is not a suggestion that abandoned or neglected children should be neglected, but that further national concentration on the welfare of the children in average poor families is also needed. There is at present a proposal before the French Chamber to extend the operation of the Roussel law of 1874, which secured some medical inspection of boarded-out infants, though this was often irregular. The proposal is to the effect that the infants of all parents in the receipt of public help, and of any other parents who may ask for it, will come within the scope of the Roussel law.

Infant mortality is excessive in France. Although it is not quite clear that the figures, owing to differences in definition of live-birth, are strictly comparable, the following rates (per 1,000 live-births) may be given:—

Years 1901–05 139
Year 1927   83

In England, in 1927, the infant death-rate was 70, in New York State 72, in Norway 48, in Germany 97. The backward position of France is further indicated by the fact that in the period 1915–20 about 23 per cent. of all the deaths of infants were caused by infantile diarrhœa. In Paris during 1905–14 one-third of the total infant mortality was due to this preventible disease.

The official organisations concerned in the protection of infant life are as follows:—

Ministère de l'Hygiène, de l'Assistance et de la Prévoyance Sociale.
Le Conseil supérieur d'Hygiène Publique de France.
Le Conseil supérieur de l'Assistance Publique.
Le Conseil supérieur de la Natalité.
Le Conseil supérieur de Protection des Enfants du premier âge.

These bodies have in the main a consultative rôle. They are related to the important voluntary body already named: *Le Comité National de l'Enfance.*

The departmental organisation is shown in the accounts of local work.

Related to these are the Consultations de Nourrisons, which are now increasingly being incorporated into Dispensaires d'Hygiène Sociale, in which may be treated, or at least advised, patients with tuberculosis, venereal disease, and sometimes cancer, as well as mothers and their infants.

Social Dispensaries.—This project of social dispensaries was begun on a considerable scale in 1923 under official auspices; and by an earlier law enacted in April 1916 their establishment was made obligatory in communes in which the death-rate had exceeded the average during five consecutive years.

The movement for the institution of these polyvalent[1] dispensaries has steadily grown; and this development is among the most hopeful of the public health movements of France.

In some areas they are still only dispensaries for tuberculosis or venereal disease, or infant consultations; and each of these needs consideration from the point of view of private and public medical practice.

We need not describe the organisations for *placement familial* or *placement collectif* of infants, which have been organised from 1874 onwards under the Roussel law. Similarly the Cantines Maternelles, Crèches, and Chambres d'Allaitement do not differ greatly from those found elsewhere. They are doing admirable work for a limited proportion of the total infants of France.

More important are the *Consultations de Nourrisons* and *Gouttes de Lait*, which give important guidance to mothers in whose care children are retained. In these, as a rule, but little medical treatment is given, and friction between private and medical practice which might follow departure from this rule has been experienced but little in France.

Similar provisions for the pre-school ages (2 to 5) scarcely exist in France on any considerable scale; and this is not surprising in view of France's unsatisfactory position as regards—

[1] By polyvalent dispensaries is meant dispensaries in which many or all diseases may be treated, for which in-patient treatment is not required.

The Medical Inspection of School Children

The low birth-rate and almost declining population of France suggests that the hygiene of childhood and of school children should form a much more prominent and active part of its public administration than it actually does.

In fact, school medical inspection is not generally organised in France. At the present time (M. Landry) in only 30 out of France's 89 départements, and in 1,693 out of its 27,000 communes, is there a service of medical inspection of schools; and even in the large cities, in which it exists, the position is usually unsatisfactory. The regulations respecting it are admirable; but only in a few cities are they even partially practised.

In the Département of the Seine, including Paris, there are numerous school medical inspectors who are part-time officers, under the guidance of Dr. L. Dufestel, who is the chief medical inspector of schools for Paris. Dr. Dufestel informed me that there are 180 such medical inspectors.

Under the regulations of the prefecture, each inspector is expected to keep to a regular time-table and record the results of his weekly visits. He directs his attention especially to sanitary conditions and to the prophylaxis of communicable diseases. He is also expected to make an individual examination of each child on his first admission to an elementary school. There is inadequate provision for informing parents of defects found at this examination. The need for further action has been realised by Dr. Dufestel and other school hygienists, but the fear of interference with the family doctor has impeded further action; and so it happens that in Paris the school doctors give statistics of the number of scholars needing spectacles or dental care, with the sole result that "These statistical reports have no other effect than to encumber the dusty portfolios of the Préfecture of the Seine" (Dr. Génévrier, in *Médicine Sociale*, 1925).

In a few cities school dispensaries have, however, been organised, often in connection with social hygiene dispensaries. Lyons is a special example of this. I have not had the opportunity of visiting its *dispensaire médico-pédagogique*, but the following particulars taken from Dr. Génévrier's article in *Médicine Sociale*, 1925, show that here some valuable medical school work is being done. The dispensary is open to all children attending the municipal schools for whom the medical inspector wishes the advice of a specialist. It has been opened because of the difficulty in securing satisfactory diagnosis and treatment for these children at hospitals. These are overburdened with patients, and prolonged waiting in promiscuous crowds has been found, as in other countries, to be very undesirable for children. In Paris, for instance, Dr. Dufestel notes that a child may have to wait three or four months before he can be operated on for adenoids.

Children are referred from the Lyons dispensary to their parents to secure the needed treatment; and it is only for indigent children that this is carried out at the dispensary.

ANTI-TUBERCULOSIS WORK

France was a pioneer in our knowledge of the pathology of tuberculosis. Villemin's epoch-making experiments, published in 1865, established the essential distinction between the virus producing this disease and the lesions produced by it; Robert Koch, by means of new and improved technique, obtaining the credit for Germany of the identification of the *corpus delicti*, the tubercle bacillus.

At an earlier period Laennec (1781–1826) had prepared the way for Villemin's researches, and had shown that every phthisis develops from tubercles, phthisis and tuberculosis in this particular being interchangeable terms.

Notwithstanding the outstanding contemporary scientific work of Calmette and other French scientists, France's practical record in the control of tuberculosis is unsatisfactory.

In 1926 there were 66,843 recorded deaths from tuberculosis in France, giving a death-rate of 1·64 per 1,000 of population. The death-rate from pulmonary tuberculosis was 1·40 per 1,000. In view of the exaggerated importance

attached to *le secret médical* in France, it is more than possible
that these figures understate the facts; and it is noteworthy
that the notification of cases of tuberculosis to the health
authority still remains optional.

In France Dr. Calmette, in 1905, initiated in Lille the
Dispensary as a means of fighting tuberculosis, his ideal
being an organisation not only for the treatment of patients,
but also for watching over their welfare, visiting them in
their homes, giving them all necessary hygienic instructions, and providing material aid when needed. Evidently
such a system, and the contemporary independent dispensary arrangements inaugurated by Dr. (now Sir Robert)
Phillip in Edinburgh, did not entirely meet the communal
needs for prophylaxis, unless associated with obligatory
notification of cases of tuberculosis by the private doctor
in attendance. In England and Scotland this was provided;
and it has become possible to make the dispensary the focus
for all hygienic measures, including systematic home visitation by public health nurses for cases of tuberculosis in
the entire community, and not merely for this disease in
dispensary patients. In France the fetish of *le secret médical*
has continued to make this in a large measure impracticable. This opposition comes much more "du bas que
du haut des corps médical", for in 1913, and again in 1919,
the Academy of Medicine has declared its endorsement of
obligatory notification of tuberculosis. There is "facultative" notification, but tuberculosis in practice is seldom
notified to the health authority.

Prior to the Great War, anti-tuberculosis work in France
was isolated and unmethodical. The establishment of the
Permanent Commission for protection against tuberculosis,
with M. Leon Bourgeois as its president, began a new era.
Legislation authorising dispensaries was passed in 1917;
but this legislation failed to provide the needed funds from
national sources, the finding of which was left to private
benefactions, aided occasionally by local governing authorities. Concerted action of the Commission headed by M.
Bourgeois with the American Commission against Tuber-

culosis and the Rockefeller Foundation enabled active work to be pushed forward, and the formation in 1919 of the Comité National de Défense Contre la Tuberculose led to organisation of measures on a national scale. This body consists of forty members, and it receives a somewhat scanty subvention from the State. Its administrative work is in liaison with the scientific studies of L'Œuvre de la

FRANCE.—ANTI-TUBERCULOSIS MEASURES (1927)

	Number of Institutions	Number of Beds	Number of Patients treated in the Year
Dispensaries	603[1]	—	186,906
Sanatoria for pulmonary tuberculosis	82	7,889	19,350
For other forms of tuberculosis	63	12,860	22,751
For all forms of tuberculosis.	5	541	1,444
Tuberculosis hospitals ..	15	3,160	8,797
Working colonies, workshop schemes, etc.	4	210	390
Preventoria	145	10,807	27,073
Open-air schools	145	3,500	16,000

[1] In 1929 this number was 640.

Tuberculose. The general character of the work of the comité is shown in the following summary, copied from the statement displayed in the entrance of its central office.

This work comprises on its social side:—

1. Technical service (technical instruction and anti-tuberculosis dispensaries).
   Various inquiries and visits.
2. Service of propaganda.
3. Service of statistics.
4. School of Visiting Nurses (250, Boulevard Raspail, Paris 14ème).

The Committee also—

Edits various publications;
Subsidises dispensaries;

Instructs on anti-tuberculosis methods;
Arranges for the placing of patients, etc.;
Is in liaison with the Ministry of Labour,
National Office of Hygiene,
Social departmental organisations and various establishments.

That much important work is now being done in France is clear from the statistical statement, shown on previous page, for which I am indebted to Dr. Humbert, the Director of the Health Division of the League of Red Cross Societies. There has been especially a great increase in the number of dispensaries and in the extent of their work. These, which were only about fifteen in 1913, have increased in 1928 to 603. The following particulars, taken from *L'Armement Anti-tuberculeuse Française* (1926), contrast the position in 1924 with that of 1918 :—

	1918	1924
Number of départements having dispensaries	6	69
Number of dispensaries	13	436
Number of new cases attending ..	7,821	107,904
Number of new cases in which tuberculosis diagnosed	2,465	43,561
Number of gratuitous consultations ..	29,106	494,278
Number of home visits	26,371	556,006

The increased activity shown above implies rapidly widening anxiety as to the prevalence of tuberculosis; doubtless, also, some influence has been exercised by the clause in the Dispensary Law of 1917 making the creation of a dispensary obligatory when the death-rate in a commune has been higher than the mean of the département during five consecutive years.

The dispensaries may be :—

(1) Public, with certain privileges, if they conform to definite rules laid down in official regulations on dispensaries. Their budget is derived from the départements and municipalities or from private resources;

(2) Private, chiefly created by mutual insurance *caisses*.

(3) Dispensaries created by public administrative bodies. These can be made compulsory by the State if during five consecutive years the mortality in a given area is higher than the average mortality in the country. The expenses of this third class of dispensaries must be borne by the municipality, with a subsidy from the State.

Relation of Tuberculosis Dispensaries to the Medical Profession. —The work of these dispensaries has been the subject of much controversy. Between 1920 and 1923 there was considerable polemic as to the tuberculosis dispensaries promoted by the Rockefeller Foundation in France. These had a highly beneficial effect in promoting anti-tuberculosis activities.

In the département of Eure-et-Loire, the number of new patients mounted up to 2,000 under American organisation, then fell when medical opposition was organised to 565, afterwards slowly increasing again (*Revue de Phthisiologie*, mars–avril 1925. M. Jacques Parisot, Nancy).

Opposition has now quieted down, and in most départements some measure of co-operation between tuberculosis dispensaries and medical syndicates has been secured. After protracted discussion it has been ruled that—

"En aucun cas, le roulement entre les médecins practiciens ne sera admis."[1]

(In no case shall doctors take turns in the medical work of the dispensary.)

Although this is so, the history of the controversy has useful lessons, inasmuch as the history of efforts at publicly organised anti-tuberculosis work repeats itself in different countries.

The medical profession of France has become organised into a Medical Syndicate or Association (Syndicat Médical),

---

[1] *Règlement Intérieur des Dispensaires antituberculeux Approuvé per le conseil de Direction du Comité National de Défense contre la Tuberculose* (17 mars, 1928), Publications of the Comité National de Défense contre la Tuberculose. Mason & Cie, Editeurs, Libraires de l'Académie de Médecine, 120. Boulevard Saint-Germain, Paris, VI, 1928.

local syndicates being affiliated to a national organisation. To this 15,000 out of the total 20,000 physicians in France (in 1926) belong. This syndicate has agitated to secure that the local syndicate shall control the appointment of the chief medical officer of each dispensary, and that part-time medical officers in the locality shall take turns in this work.

The contention of the Syndicat Médical has been that the dispensary should not be a complete organism by itself, medically and for home visits, but that it should be under the control of the family doctor of each patient. This contention unfortunately ignored the fact that a large proportion of dispensary patients have no family doctor; and that in many cases attended by such a doctor, he is too busy or too preoccupied to undertake the hygienic work involved.

The Syndicat Médical further urged that the administrative type of dispensary rests on a fundamentally erroneous assumption, viz. that it is possible to separate prophylaxis from therapeutics. With this view there must be a large measure of agreement, for treatment widely interpreted is perhaps the most valuable means of prophylaxis at our disposal for tuberculosis. But what treatment? Apart from such special measures as the administration of tuberculin or the treatment of artificial pneumothorax, the chief form of treatment at the dispensary consists in arranging for the patient's institutional treatment when this is indicated, for the hygienic control of coughing and spitting, and for the provision of separate sleeping accommodation and adequate nutrition and nursing at home. These can be arranged through the dispensary; they are commonly neglected in cases suitable for dispensary care, unless the dispensary organisation is utilised.

This contention, furthermore, neglects the important ancillary functions of the dispensary: the search for undetected cases of tuberculosis, the removal of insanitary and dusty conditions, domiciliary or occupational, the attempt to control alcoholism, etc.

Other objections to the official type of dispensary have

been that the private practitioner is superseded, and that the health visitors often do not give advice in accordance with that of the private doctor. These objections evidently can be met, while at the same time the consultant services of the dispensary, especially in the diagnosis of doubtful cases by X-rays or otherwise, can be made to add greatly to the efficiency of private medical practice.

One objection, which bulked largely in the minds of French physicians, will not be sympathetically regarded by most physicians of other countries. It is that the dispensary attempts to utilise the medical profession in its effort to establish medical police supervision over consumptives. This is another form of statement of objection to any infringement of *le secret médical* (page 86). There must, in accordance with this view, be no compulsory notification of cases of tuberculosis, and it is even doubted whether death certificates should reveal the real cause of death, if any direct or indirect reflection on the family of the deceased is implied in the certificate, as, for example, when there has been cancer or tuberculosis or syphilis. This objection on the part of organised private physicians appears to me to be an unanswerable reason for promoting to the utmost the resort of consumptives to dispensaries. The point can be illustrated from an article by Dr. Evrot in *Revue de Phthisiologie Médico-Sociale* (January–February 1924). In that year 50,000 tuberculous patients were being treated in the dispensaries, of whom 12,000 were bacilliferous. Dr. Evrot pertinently asks, were these patients previously the subject of any active domiciliary surveillance? There is little doubt that in most instances the answer must be an emphatic negative.

Among the further contentions of the syndicate was the demand that any doctor elected by the syndicate should take charge at the dispensary, without guarantee as to his special experience and skill in tuberculosis. Another demand was that payment should be on the basis of number of consultations at each attendance. It is not surprising that Dr. E. Rist should state in the same *Revue* that while cordially acknowledging the work of many private doctors, syndicalist or non-syndicalist—

I cannot conceal this truth of experience that the gravest obstacle to the efficient work of the dispensary consists in the ignorance, incompetence, carelessness, absence of all social sense which characterise a minority of practitioners, syndicalist or not.

One has to struggle daily against errors of diagnosis, of therapeutics, of prophylaxis, ignoring absolutely social conditions and the true interests of patients and their contacts.

The *Revue* already mentioned gives statements by Professor Leon Bernard, Dr. E. Rist, and others, setting out the points at issue from the standpoint of the Comité National de Défense contre la Tuberculose. The burden of these contributions is a contrast between the dispensaries of the comité and those of the "type syndicaliste". Dr. Calmette signs a preliminary statement on behalf of the Comité National as to the measures of collaboration between the dispensaries and the medical profession which are recommended by the comité to all local organisations:—

1. There should be periodic reunions at each dispensary at which the medical officer of the dispensary and the chief health visitor should confer with a representative of the local medical syndicate.

2. The same practice should hold good for the collective dispensaries of each region.

3. The staff of the dispensary should be at the disposal of the local physicians.

   (*a*) To enquire into any act of the personnel of dispensaries which is contrary to the legitimate interests of physicians;

   (*b*) To convey to each physician full information respecting any patient sent by him to the dispensary; and

   (*c*) To examine the sputum of any patient who cannot attend the dispensary.

No definite agreement appears to have been reached on these lines; but the open agitation against the dispensaries has subsided.

There can be little doubt that in the present year, 1929, the Syndicat Médical would state their case differently from what is indicated above; that they would now agree that their privileged position as family physicians carries serious social responsibilities; and that, furthermore, dispensaries have been able to render them valuable help in securing for their patients the advantages of skilled diagnosis and of the special treatment in institutions and elsewhere which their patients require.

As an illustration of the extent to which co-operation has been organised may be given the following summarised particulars of the Contractual Entente proposed between L'Œuvre Anti-tuberculeuse and the Federation of Medical Syndicates of the Department of Bouches-du-Rhône (October 1925).

1. *Rôle of Dispensaries and Doctors.*—(*a*) The public dispensaries of social hygiene and of protection against tuberculosis are specially concerned, in terms of the law of 1916 (titre I, 1st article) with anti-tuberculous education, with giving advice on prophylaxis and hygiene, and with obtaining for tuberculous patients admission into hospitals, sanatoria, and other places for treatment; also to ensure for the public a service for the disinfection of contaminated linen, articles, places, and rooms. No treatment is to be given at the dispensary. In certain special cases a service for care and for the distribution of medicaments may be organised, but it is understood that this only applies to cases where the patient is recognised as being necessitous, and, in terms of the law of 1916, "in accord with the local or regional services of hygiene and of assistance", that is after agreement with the representatives of the L'Assistance Médicale Gratuite and the Federation of Medical Syndicates of the department.

(*b*) Medical practitioners are the indispensable active collaborators of every anti-tuberculosis organisation. Their rôle is to attend tuberculous patients who come to them, and to communicate with the dispensary in regard to those whose illness and material situation appear to the doctors to justify the intervention of L'Œuvre Anti-tuberculeuse.

2. *Liaison between Dispensaries and Medical Practitioners.*— The following measures enable the conditions of the liaison between the dispensary and the practising doctor to be regulated.

(*a*) *Patients sent by Doctors.*—Every doctor may avail himself of the services of dispensaries for a diagnosis or its confirmation. In this case the patient is submitted to a *complete* examination, carried out by all the scientific methods of investigation. This is not practicable in isolated dispensaries, e.g. those not having facilities for radioscopy.

On the other hand the patient ought to have his name registered at the dispensary; he thus secures, with the approval of his doctor, the prophylactic action of the dispensary which follows on registration.

The complete result of examinations conducted at the dispensary should be transmitted to the medical practitioner in the form of a confidential "fiche de liaison".

(*b*) *Patients who have come spontaneously and those sent to the Dispensary.*—The dispensary will make inquiries as to whether the patient has a private doctor; the name and address of the latter should be noted in the *fiche*, and the dispensary doctor should notify the private doctor, and place at his disposal the "fiche de liaison" giving the results of clinical radiological and bacteriological examinations.

(*c*) *Patients confined to bed notified by Doctors.*—By agreement with these, such patients will benefit by the prophylactic services and the assistance of the dispensary on whose roll their names are entered.

(*d*) The dispensary will advise doctors of any decision as to the removal of their patients to establishments for cure or isolation, and will also notify them of their return to their families.

3. *The Rôle of Visiting Nurses* (*Infirmières-visiteuses*).—These will try to establish relations with the doctor in charge in order usefully to fulfill their rôle, which is purely hygienic. They will refrain from all therapeutic initiative; only in exceptional and urgent cases may they "donner de soins", and then always subject to notification to the doctor in charge.

4. *Liaison in the Conseil d'Administration.*—To ensure a permanent liaison between L'Œuvre and the Syndicates, the Conseil d'Administration will include the president of the Federation of Medical Syndicates of Bouches-du-Rhône and a representative of the Medical Syndicate of Marseilles among its official members. The last-named will be appointed by the federation for two years and eligible for re-election.

5. *Nomination of Dispensary Doctors.*—The nomination of dispensary doctors will be made by the Departmental Committee from a list of the Medical Commission of the Œuvre, to which have been added for this purpose the delegates of the Federation of the Medical Syndicates of the Bouches-du-Rhône.

The present agreement has been concluded for an experimental year. It is renewable by tacit consent.

Signed by   Marseilles, *October* 26, 1925.
Vice-President of   Président de la Fédération des
L'Œuvre anti-   Syndicats médicaux des Bouches.
tuberculeuse.   du-Rhône.

In the Département of Meurthe-et-Moselle a close entente has been secured between the official Office d'Hygiène Sociale and L'Association Syndicale des Médicins of the Département. (See *L'Organisation de la Lutte Anti-Tuberculeuse*, J. Parisot, 1928.) In the year 1920 only one tuberculosis patient was sent to the tuberculosis dispensary by a private doctor; in 1927 the proportion so sent was 90 per cent. of all known patients. In this département also there is one hospital bed for tuberculous patients per 1,080 inhabitants, or 1·6 beds for each death from tuberculosis.

Infirmières Hospitalières.—A great difficulty in securing good anti-tuberculosis work has been the fact that before the war there were few trained nurses in France. When some 13,000 nuns were discharged from the hospitals of France, there were very few competent women to take their place.

After the war many war nurses became public health nurses; but home visiting by public health nurses is still exceptional, except for patients attending dispensaries, and often it is very incomplete for them.

Gradually the position in this respect is improving. Three diplomas are now given to nurses—one for infirmary nurses, one showing competence in infant hygiene and tuberculosis, and one for hospitals. A council has been formed called Le Conseil de Perfectionnement des Ecoles Infirmières (1922), analogous to the English College of Nursing.

In Paris, Bordeaux, Lyons, Nantes, and Rheims there already exist schools at which infirmières-visiteuses are trained for their work in infant-school hygiene and in tuberculosis work.

Budget for Tuberculosis.—With increasing anti-tuberculosis work, financial expenditure in France for this purpose has greatly increased. Thus the subsidies of the State for 1929 amount approximately to 73,000,000 French francs, against 63 millions in 1928. The chief items of these subsidies[1] are :—

		Francs
(a) Organisation of dispensaries; bacteriological laboratories, child welfare, Œuvre Grancher, and similar	.. ..	18,000,000
(b) Construction or adaptation of tuberculosis sanatoria	.. ..	25,000,000
(c) Creation and transformation of preventoria	..	7,000,000
(d) Individual assistance to tuberculous patients	..	12,000,000
(e) Exceptional contribution of the State for the creation of villages for gassed tuberculous ex-soldiers	.. ..	500,000

The sum spent by the State approximates frs. 1.75 *per capita*.

The sum spent by municipalities, départements, or private organisations varies greatly according to the region. It is stated, for instance, that in the Département de Finistère nearly one-third of the sum expended is provided by private initiative alone (fêtes, bazaars, voluntary subscriptions), the rest being raised by State or municipality; in other départements the sum paid by municipalities or préfectures comes near to 50 per cent. of the State Budget. The local proportion is very likely never greater and often smaller than this. It is in the Département de la Seine that the greatest effort is made against tuberculosis, the conditions appearing to be particularly favourable through the creation of an autonomous "Office d'Hygiène Sociale de la Seine". The sum spent in this Département *per capita* for the anti-tuberculosis movement is frs. 4.75.

Among the voluntary contributions may be quoted the product of the Christmas Seal launched on the American plan, which in 1928 brought in more than frs. 18,000,000 for the whole of France. This money is spent by the local branches of the Comité National de Défense contre la

[1] In the French Budget for 1930, item (a) has become 22 millions, item (b) 40 millions, and item (c) 10 millions.

Tuberculose in the départements where the money has been raised, a small percentage (approximately 5 per cent.) being kept by the Central Committee for general administration.

M. Tardieu, in September 1929, brought before the French Chamber a proposal to spend 400 million francs in the course of the next five years, and to provide at once 20,000 additional beds for the tuberculous. It is intended also to spend a further 300 million francs in the same period on general hospitals.

ANTI-VENEREAL WORK

As in other countries, the Great War has been followed in France by increased efforts to diminish the prevalence of syphilis and gonorrhœa.

The Commission on the Prophylaxis of Venereal Diseases estimated that one-tenth of the French population are attacked by syphilis, that it causes annually 20,000 deaths of infants between the sixth month of gestation and three days after birth, that it also causes 40,000 abortions each year, and is responsible annually for the deaths of at least 60,000 persons.

The central organisations concerned with the struggle against venereal diseases are six in number, the first-named below being official, the others entirely or in part voluntary in character.

1. The central service of prophylaxis of venereal diseases is attached to the Ministry of Assistance and Public Health.

It has a small personnel, which directs the struggle, visits clinics and other organisations, and tries to establish liaison between these.

2. The National Office of Social Hygiene is a semi-official organisation (see pages 54 and 69). Its venereal section is directed by Dr. Cavaillon, whose work, *Le Bilan de la Syphilis*, 1928, gives particulars of anti-venereal work throughout France.

3. The Commission on Prophylaxis of Venereal Disease is a consultative body.

4. The Prophylactic Institute, directed by Dr. Vernes, has organised many dispensaries, at which a constant serological control of treatment is maintained (methode de Vernes). In ten years 900,000 consultations have been held at the institute.

5. The National League against the Venereal Peril.

6. The French Society of Sanitary and Moral Prophylaxis makes studies and promotes propaganda by its affiliated society, the Committee of Feminine Education.

In the départements anti-venereal work is frequently conducted by the departmental services, through its medical inspectors. The préfet fixes the budget available for this purpose, made up out of sums voted by the Conseil Général and subsidies from the Central Government. The work may be attached to the Public Department of Social Hygiene.

Sometimes local organisations exist of a non-official character. At present there are fifty-one departmental organisations. In the remaining départements, with four exceptions, there are autonomous anti-venereal services.

Anti-syphilitic dispensaries have been opened in nearly all urban centres with a population exceeding 10,000. In great towns these are attached to the dermato-syphilographic services of the medical faculties or schools of medicine.

In the case of subsidised dispensaries, the Minister only gives subsidies when competent specialists are in charge.

The dispensaries are maintained in varying proportions by the commune, the département, and (or) the Ministry of Health and Assistance. The Central Ministry as a minimum always supplies the specific medicaments.

Private practitioners of medicine may be enabled to treat venereal patients at the public charge, subject to regulations. The Ministry can then pay the doctor, supply specific drugs, and pay the pharmacist for other drugs.

Inquiries are made as to the patient's ability to pay, but this control is not very strict.

In 1916 the State gave 200,000 francs for subsidies to

40 services; and in 1926 it gave 9,650,000 francs to 893 services.

Recently special anti-syphilitic clinics have been opened for mothers and infants; and at present 281 of the services for mothers and infants have special facilities for anti-syphilitic treatment.

Special services, 138 in number according to M. Landry, have been arranged for the treatment of venereal disease in prisons, by co-operation between the Ministries of Justice and Health.

There are twenty-nine central laboratories for serological examinations, and many others are proposed.

Cavaillon, after careful inquiries, considers that syphilis has decreased in France, and thinks that this decrease can be expressed in terms of the decline in number of still-births.

In 1912 still-births numbered 43·3 per 1,000 total births.
In 1916 still-births numbered 48·3 per 1,000 total births.
In 1925 still-births numbered 39·4 per 1,000 total births
In 1926 still-births numbered 38·5 per 1,000 total births.
In 1927 still-births numbered 37·5 per 1,000 total births.

The national budget for 1929 for anti-venereal work was 11 million francs. This was divided among 1,349 services.

MEDICAL SYNDICALISM IN FRANCE

In 1884 professional syndicalism, i.e. combined action for occupational protection, was legalised in France. Medical syndicates had been initiated as early as 1881. In 1913 there were 138 local medical syndicates with some 7,000 members; in 1928 these societies had multiplied and their membership amounted to 16,000 among the 28,000 total doctors in France. It is noticeable that more than a third of the doctors remain outside these organisations. It may be added here that in 1901 France had one doctor to 2,335 inhabitants, and that in 1928 there were 28,380 doctors to a population of 39,300,000, or one doctor to 1,400 inhabitants. In Paris and the Département of the Seine the number was one doctor to 723 inhabitants.

The activities of medical syndicates have been directed to secure satisfactory conditions of medical work from mutual sickness insurance societies, and are now concentrated on the problems of a French national system of compulsory sickness insurance. They have also been concerned with protecting the confidential relationship between doctor and patient against "third parties", whether these be courts of law, insurance authorities, or public health authorities who are interested in the prevention and treatment of disease. There is a tangle of ethical and economic factors from which France is only very gradually releasing itself.

Le Secret Médical

The strict preservation of the cherished confidential relation of doctor to patient has been rendered increasingly difficult by modern life. In recent years the intimacy of this relationship has been relaxed by the more elaborate consultative diagnosis necessitated by the progress of medicine. Examinations of pathological material from patients, references to consultants, hospital treatment, all alike make strict retention of the older view as to *le secret médical* increasingly difficult for both patient and doctor.

The medical profession in France has always objected to certification of causes of death of deceased patients. This is not safeguarded against official inquisitiveness, as it is in Switzerland. Even now this certification cannot be said to be as complete and accurate in France as in some other European countries.

The law of July 1895, providing for Assistance Médicale Gratuite for the Destitute, necessitated medical certification to the mayoralty and was a further encroachment on the assumed sacredness of the relation between doctor and patient. Furthermore, administrative delays in paying doctors for their gratuitous help often occurred, especially for attendance on accouchements, and the need for combined action of syndicated doctors grew.

Legislation as to industrial accidents raised similar

problems. By the law of 1898 the employer is responsible for all accidents, and medical certification of these has been beset with difficulties. In all these cases the individual doctor and the individual patient no longer occupy an exclusively confidential relationship, but a "third party" has become concerned, whose encroachments on the personal nexus cannot be successfully resisted. At the present time difficulties are being intensively realised in the current proposals for national sickness insurance in France (page 90).

Apart from sickness insurance, which will be separately considered, the increased interest and activity of the central and local governing authorities of France in the prevention and treatment of disease have been a chief factor in increasing syndical medical activity. This in part, but not chiefly, is due to the encroachment on the confidential relationship of doctor and patient. As already seen, syndicates in some départements have demanded that infant consultations, dispensaries, and school medical work shall be conducted by the practising doctors in a given community in an arranged rota, a proposal which—while it may assuage medical susceptibilities—is found in nearly every instance to be injurious to the efficiency of the organisation. There has been much controversy and friction between "professors of philanthropy", "officials", "medical pontiffs" on the one hand, and "practiciens" on the other. Official dispensaries have been described as merely the façade of a building, the rest of which is lacking; and it has been claimed, for instance, in the Département of the Seine, that the organisation of social medicine should be entrusted to medical syndicates.

For infectious diseases it has been partially accepted by the French medical profession that the public interest requires their notification to a responsible public authority; though for tuberculosis this notification still remains facultative. The view in favour of compulsory notification has been officially endorsed by the Conseil d'Etat, which, reporting to the French Ministry on July 20, 1928, recommended abrogation of Article 378 of the Penal Code, and endorsed the view that medical secrecy is not obligatory for contagious diseases, the social interest being greater than the individual.

A somewhat similar difficulty has arisen in regard to visits by infirmières-visiteuses to homes in which a birth had occurred. During the war the American Red Cross organised in Lyons a system for obtaining a list of births occurring in the 7th arrondissement of that city. The mayor supplied this list daily to the child welfare workers in this district. The visitors were well received and were most useful in promoting personal hygiene and in bringing parents into touch with public assistance when this was needed.

A similar attempt by an American organisation was made in 1918 in the 14th arrondissement of Paris. For six months the local mayor supplied the list of births, and visits to the homes were made. Then objection was raised that the giving of the lists involved a breach of confidential information and the work ceased, except when parents expressed a wish to be visited.

The impossibility of adhering to the older conception of *le secret médical* is further illustrated by the fact that a medical certificate to the mayoralty is a condition of securing the monthly bonus of money or gifts of milk for suckling mothers (see page 52).

Much progress has already been made in adjusting the difficulties illustrated above. The current agitation on national sickness insurance, discussed on page 90 *et seq.*, will necessarily have a determining influence on the general methods of co-operation which must emerge (see also page 96).

VOLUNTARY SICKNESS INSURANCE IN FRANCE

Although France is only now coming into line with other European countries which have adopted compulsory national systems of sickness and invalidity insurance, it has already many societies giving somewhat similar benefits on mutual and voluntary lines. The following figures are taken from the report of the International Labour Office on Voluntary Sickness Insurance (Geneva, 1927). They give statistics for the year 1924. These societies are of three kinds: *free societies*, which are independent of any public control; *approved societies*, subject to a certain measure of supervision by State authorities; and *societies of recognised*

	Number of Societies	Number of Members	
		Honorary	Full
A. FREE SOCIETIES.			
1. Societies engaged in sickness insurance .	1,536	21,830	173,958
2. Societies engaged in Sickness Insurance and Pensions Insurance	186	5,669	31,149
3. Societies engaged in Maternity Insurance	1	33	216
B. APPROVED AND RECOGNISED SOCIETIES.			
1. Societies engaged in Sickness Insurance.	7,037	137,882	1,098,380
2. Societies engaged in Sickness Insurance and Pensions Insurance	8,053	325,624	1,398,683
3. Societies engaged in Maternity Insurance	91	19,694	127,879
C. SCHOOL SOCIETIES ..	1,883	30,861	772,082
Totals	18,787	4,143,940	

public utility, subject to still stricter supervision. The two last-named classes enjoy certain financial privileges and may receive State subsidies.

Further particulars concerning these voluntary organisations are given in the official report already quoted.

Notwithstanding the large membership shown in the preceding figures, it cannot be said that these voluntary sickness societies have met with great success. The payment to doctors has been too small, and the encouragement of preventive medicine nil. Whether the projected National Insurance for Sickness will succeed remains to be seen. At present (1929) it is only a "project," and so far no funds have been allotted for the purpose. From preliminary statements it appears that the cost of the very elaborate benefits proposed to be conferred has been underestimated.

Reference may be made here to an admirable attempt, which has had only very limited success. This is—

La Mutualité Maternelle, founded in Paris in 1891 for the wives of workpeople in the Département of the Seine. This has spread into the provinces. Since 1920, in addition to insuring help for the mother and infant, medical consultations during pregnancy and lactation have also been organised by the society. The charges made for insurance do not suffice for adequate aid to the beneficiaries.

COMPULSORY SICKNESS INSURANCE IN FRANCE

This is a post-bellum development, and doubtless has been expedited by the fact that the newly annexed provinces of Alsace and Lorraine already were deeply involved in the German National System of Sickness Insurance. The new law for sickness insurance is dated April 5, 1928, and the history of its official incubation dates from March 1921, when the Minister of Labour introduced a Bill on the subject embodying the result of the deliberations of a technical commission appointed in 1919.

The proposals were referred for further consideration, and in April 1924 they were agreed to by the Chamber of Deputies unanimously and without discussion. The Senate, on receiving the proposals, referred them to its Commission of Hygiene, which consulted interested societies and circles, and then, through Dr. Chauveau, its president, put forward proposals more succinct and otherwise modified from those to which the Chamber of Deputies had agreed. Towards the end of 1925 the Minister of Labour appointed a further representative commission to report on the report of the Senatorial Commission. This second report was presented by Dr. Chauveau in November 1926. While this second commission was sitting, collateral commissions were at work from the point of view of commerce, agriculture, public works, finance, legislation, and administration; and following on these a third and supplementary report was made by Dr. Chauveau.

This was discussed by the Senate on June 9, 1927, and afterwards, during thirteen sittings of the Senate, 154 amendments being presented. The Senate adopted its final proposals on July 7, 1927, by 269 votes to 2.

These proposals were referred to the Chamber of Deputies on July 13, 1927, and were made the subject of a two-volumed report by Drs. Grinda and Antonelli. Their discussion by the Deputies began on March 8, 1928. After four sittings devoted to general discussion, the seventy-four sections of the Bill were approved in two sittings without any modification of its text as transmitted from the Senate. The impending end of the session and an impending general election appear to have been the reason for this hurried action; but it is unfortunate that the many criticisms which had been voiced within and without the Chamber were not adequately considered.[1] It is especially noteworthy that while the Bill was with the Senate no special committee representing the medical profession had been officially concerned with its proposals. That there were, and continue to be, many objections from the medical profession will be seen shortly.

First, however, we may state the main provisions of the Bill which relate to problems of medical care.

Proposals of the Act.—The essential point in social insurance is to give some guarantee against social risk. It is to be distinguished from professional risk, which is largely a

---

[1] Some of the particulars here given are well set out in *Qu'est-ce que les Assurances sociales* by H. Solus, Professor of Law in the University of Poitiers.

problem of accident insurance. The intention of social insurance is to supplant charity and to supersede it by foresight working by means of compulsory insurance. As stated eloquently in the parliamentary discussion on insurance, the French worker is "encore un isolé", still the afflicted victim of industrial uncertainty "le cauchemar de lendemain".

The new law proposes to insure against the following risks:—

Sickness,
Maternity,
Invalidity,
Old Age,
Death,
Unemployment.

In the words of M. Fallières, the Minister of Labour, it is intended also to be a bond of union and concord between master and men and between these and the State. A delay of one year was arranged for the necessary executive arrangements, an interval which has already passed, without much further progress being made. The resources of French finance are heavily involved in the scheme.

The law provides that the Départements of Haut-Rhin, Bas-Rhin, and la Moselle shall be separately treated until the necessary adjustments of the former Alsace and Lorraine can be made. Meanwhile the domination of the German medical profession by the German societies has been avoided, it is believed, in the provisions of the French law.

Every employed person, male or female, with a total annual salary not exceeding 18,000 francs is included in the scheme, except certain employees of the State, State railways, and miners, for whom provision is otherwise made.

The limit of 18,000 francs is not a fixed sum. It is increased by 2,000 francs for each infant after the first. "Infants" are counted up to the age of sixteen years. If there is no infant in charge of the insured, compulsory insurance only applies up to a salary of 15,000 francs.

The département is the unit of administrative organisation of social insurance, and in each département its execution is entrusted to a single departmental caisse or insurance society and to "primary caisses". Each of these is constituted in accordance with the law of April 1, 1898, on Mutual Insurance Societies. All persons liable to be insured must be insured in the département in which they work. The departmental caisse will supervise the primary caisses, the number of which is unlimited, controlled only by local initiative and needs. Thus the insured can group themselves by locality or by occupation as they choose. Generally this grouping will be in the hands of societies already existing under the law of 1898. The work of the caisses is under a double control, that of the National Office of Social Insurances and the complementary control exercised by the Ministries of Labour and of Finance.

The departmental caisse comprises eighteen members, of whom six are designated by the Departmental Union of Societies of Mutual Aid, six by Agricultural Mutual Aid Societies, and six by the syndicates of employees. The administration of the primary caisses is in the hands of the body organising them.

The State is regarded as having fulfilled its obligation in social insurance by the provision of medical and other aid for the destitute; and the cost of social insurance for others is borne by employees and workers in equal parts. The payment of contributions by the employer is regarded as justified by his presumed obligation to make good his human material, as he does other parts of his outfit, both economic and humanitarian motives demanding this aid.

The contribution of the employer is 5 per cent., and of the worker 5 per cent. of the total salary of the latter.

No lower age limit is fixed for the commencement of insurance; but payments cease at the age of 60, when an old age pension becomes payable. If a worker continues to work at a higher age, he is exempt from wage deductions, but is not eligible for sickness money benefits.

Sickness Benefits.—These consist of medical treatment and an allowance of half the wages. Medical treatment is given also to the insured person's wife and children under 16 years old.

There is no limitation of disease, such as occurs in the English insurance law, in accordance with which the treatment given to the insured person must be within the competence of a general medical practitioner of average ability. Complete medical, surgical, and pharmaceutical treatment, and, in addition, preventive treatment, are included. Thus the cost of hospital treatment and of treatment at cure stations is included.

By Article 6 (1) of the Law the insured is entitled to consultations and treatment in the dispensaries, clinics, establishments for cure and prevention which belong to the insurance caisse with which he is insured.

The free choice of doctor was much discussed in the Senate, and finally [Article 4 (2)] it was enacted that—

Medical consultations are given at the doctor's house, except when the patient cannot leave his home. For visits at home, the insured is limited to doctors or midwives of the commune in which he resides, or of the nearest available commune. When the insured desires to consult another doctor, or, in general, any doctor whose fees are higher than those of the local tariffs, the excess of cost for such a consultation will be paid by the insured.

By Article 4 (4) it is enacted that—

The enrolments for domiciliary treatment and for hospital and other treatment shall be in accordance with agreements between the local medical syndicate and the insurance caisse.

It is required that these contracts shall be submitted for arbitration to a special Tripartite Commission [Article 7 (3)], composed in equal numbers of representatives of the caisses, of professional groups, and of the office of Social Insurances.

In practice the medical syndicates will act for practitioners in negotiating with the representatives of the caisses as to the conditions of medical service. If the insured person consults a doctor who has not agreed to the tariff arranged by the medical syndicate, any excess of charge by this doctor must be defrayed by the insured. To a certain extent this proviso limits the free choice of doctor.

To avoid abuse of medical aid, it is provided [Article 4 (5)] that the share of the insured in the cost of medical care and drugs shall amount to 15 to 20 per cent. This proviso is made experimental for a period of two years.

Sickness is considered to date from the day of the first medical consultation, and sickness allowance begins five days later. When the patient enters a hospital, a reduced money allowance is made according to the size of his family.

The administrative control of insurance is in the hands of the caisses; technical control of the quality of the professional work is exercised by the professional syndicates on their own initiative or on the demand of the caisse.

Maternity Benefits.—These consist of medical care, of a semi-salary, and of primes d'allaitement. The wage-earning insured woman is entitled (Article 9) to the following benefits, and the wife of an insured person to some of them.

1. During pregnancy and for six months afterwards, each of these is entitled to medical and pharmaceutical care, on the lines already set out.

2. For six weeks before and six weeks after accouchement an insured woman is entitled to half her ordinary wages, so long as she abstains from any salaried work.

3. If any pathological conditions supervene, the rules of sickness insurance apply for insured women.

4. Every insured woman who suckles her infant is entitled during lactation and for a period up to a year to a special monthly allowance of 100 francs during the first two months, of 75 francs from the third to the fifth month, of 50 francs in the sixth month, and of 25 francs from the seventh to the ninth month, and then of 15 francs each month from the tenth to the twelfth.

5. If she is unable to suckle her infant, and this fact is certified by the doctor, an insured woman can still receive her "bons de lait," to the extent of not more than two-thirds of the "prime d'allaitement."

6. The above payments are subject to home visits on behalf of the caisse and to regular attendance at the maternal consultations of infant hygiene centres.

I do not propose to summarise the clauses of the law relating to invalidity and the legal and administrative sections. What has already been given suffices to show the general character of the new French law as bearing on the relation between the doctor and his patient and between the doctor and the insurance caisses.

Whether financial stress will permit the complete carrying out of the law remains to be seen. Meanwhile it is of profound social interest that France has now come into the rank of those European countries which are providing medical attendance for a very large share of the total population on the basis of contracts between insurance societies (caisses) and medical syndicates, or on the basis (as in Hungary) of contracts between governmental insurance bodies and medical syndicates.

LE SECRET MÉDICAL (*continued*)

Evidently these developments affect momentously the problems associated with "le secret medical" already partially discussed (page 86). They have been widely canvassed by the French medical profession, and heated discussions have been followed by resolutions which in English parlance may be called "die-hard". Thus the physicians of the Département du Nord have affirmed that the new insurance law is incompatible with the honest and proper practice of medicine and have decided that they "refuse their collaboration to the Insurance Law as it stands at present".

At a recent meeting of medical syndicates in France the following resolution was passed:—

Respect for medical secrecy constitutes for the doctor an absolute rule in every circumstance.

Past experience shows that the violation of this secret has not produced favourable results in law and regulations, and confirms the justice of this fundamental principle in medicine.

The medical body, therefore, demands not only that medical secrecy shall be rigorously respected in future laws and regulations, but also that the laws and regulations now in force shall, as far as possible, be revised to the same effect.

There is needed study, both by legislative and administrative bodies, of means for defending the public health without violation of medical secrecy.

In view of such a pronounced expression of medical opinion, it is not unlikely that before the Act is brought into operation some further modifications in it will be made.

The fact that medical certificates come into the hands of the officials of insurance caisses is a chief stumbling-block to medical endorsement of national sickness insurance. The medical syndicates of France have affirmed that they cannot collaborate in the social insurance law unless this assures absolute medical secrecy, "which ought not to be violated directly or indirectly".

It is also claimed that giving the medical certificate to the patient instead of to the caisse—thus making the patient responsible for publication—is an indirect violation of secrecy; that, in short, the patient's consent does not relieve the doctor from secrecy. This contention throws back the argument on the point whether a State has the right, through its representatives in Parliament, to compel a large section of the total population to contribute compulsorily to provision against sickness. This need not be debated here, but such an enactment having been made, the insured person's interests evidently necessitate accurate and carefully safeguarded medical certification to the caisse administering insurance. The doctor, I think, cannot continue to regard himself as compelled to defend a patient against certification of sickness to a third party, when the national legislature has imposed on each worker a compulsion which necessitates this certification.

That this position is untenable is illustrated by the admission in practice that infringements of medical secrecy are legitimate when demanded by the public interests; and it would appear that certification of births, of deaths and their causes, of occupational diseases, and of accidents already come into this category. It can seldom, if ever, be shown in such cases that the special interest of the person certified or of his relatives need necessarily be injuriously affected by the certification. The efforts of public authorities are almost uniformly devoted to the prevention of this possibility; abuses when they occur can be remedied; and nearly every suggestible evil ceases when such certification becomes a general practice.

There can, I think, be little doubt that ere long the older and more rigid doctrine of medical secrecy will be modified in France to enable social insurance to have a fair prospect of working success.

My own opinion on this discussion can be stated in the words of Professor Barthélemy, a distinguished French jurist, and of Dr. Rist, a distinguished physician in Paris. Professor Barthélemy very properly says medical secrecy paralyses justice ("La règle du secret énerve la justice"); and Dr. Rist states his conviction that "the doctrine of absolute medical secrecy supplies a means of escaping cases of conscience, of declining responsibility, and of washing one's hands of the most obvious duties". This appears to be in his view the true reason for the passionate adhesion of so many doctors to this doctrine.[1]

Further Medical Objections to Sickness Insurance.—In the above brief summary I have not attempted to describe the general objections to social insurance felt by a large section of the French medical profession. I must content myself with a brief statement of these.

The view is entertained by many that sickness insurance means that in future doctors will cease to have patients and only consider diseases. This by implication suggests that the patients treated in public hospitals and under L'Assistance Publique fail generally to receive that humane care from doctors which is the lot of private patients. Is either side of this statement, whether it relates to private or to public patients, the general truth? And is it seriously contended that whole-time official doctors—not chosen directly by the individual patient—as a class do not give humane treatment to their patients?

When Dr. P. Guérin[2] inveighs against the scandalous overcrowding of tuberculous patients in hospitals, the inadequacy of sanatoria, the excessive infant mortality, and

[1] Quoted by Dr. P. Guérin in *L'Etat contre le Médecin*, Paris, 1929.
[2] *L'Etat contre le Médecin*, Paris, 1929.

other evidences of lack of personal and communal hygiene in France, one can heartily agree; and we may even agree that insurance to obtain medical treatment is a poor substitute for the public health measures which ought to have preceded and which we hope may accompany this insurance. But it must also be stated that the same physicians who object to sickness insurance have also objected to public health work whenever it impinges on the work of the private physician.

The contention that insurance means the "negation of effort", and that France will soon be divided into two halves, one-half assisting, the other being assisted, strikes deeply; for a great danger in official insurance is the tendency to make claims unduly or even unfairly on the funds to which the insured person has contributed. The cultivation of the fraternal conscience which was marked in the older English friendly societies, and which is less apparent as a rule in official societies, is a great need of all forms of social insurance. Is it hopeless to anticipate the growth of such a conscience?

Meanwhile a further danger of social insurance is the creation of a hypertrophic official class, excessive in numbers, and possessed of dangerous financial and political power. On this point France's fears may be compared with the experience of some of the European countries which is summarised in this volume and in my Vol. I.

The cost of excessive officialism and of undue claims on the insurance funds is borne to the extent of one-half by the insured person himself, and the other half is an overhead expense of industry. When these points are generally realised, employers and employed alike will increasingly take action to prevent the frequent abuses of social insurance, and in this work will seek for the active co-operation of the doctors attending the insured sick.

In all countries insurance against sickness has hitherto been associated with the creation of much artificial sickness. It has been said that every well man is a self-forgetting patient. When insured, and there is a prospect of sick allowances, too often he ceases to be self-forgetting. Here a distinction is needed. If sickness, as the result of sickness insurance, is recognised earlier and scientifically treated, certain and adequate treatment is all to the good; such treatment becomes a valuable aid to personal hygiene. But it must be admitted that there is also a frequent failure in the will to keep well, and in the will to get well when ill, among insured persons. Will the average individual conscience rise above this persistent temptation?

As bearing on the creation of excessive claims for sickness, I may quote a letter sent me by a physican of repute in Paris, who is not engaged in private medical practice, and who evidently does not share the views in favour of direct payment in proportion to work done, vehemently held by medical syndicates in France. He says:—

The German system of payment of doctors for actual visits or consultations, proposed by the French law, soon leads to a mechanisation of medical treatment, since the common interests of physician and patient encourage prolongation of treatment and multiplication of visits, for the ensurement of money benefits. The English system (of average capitation payments, whether ill or not) tends much more to interest the physician in public health and personal hygiene, and thus towards the diminution of sickness. The establishment of hospitals and clinics by insurance societies conducted by experts ought, notwithstanding the adverse criticisms of their operation, to form a corrective to individual medical attendance under the German system.

As bearing on this point, M. Cazeneuve has recently quoted German experience in 1926 to the effect that there was control of the condition of 1,259,016 patients in 778 caisses, having altogether 7,918,412 members, with the result that 56·5 per cent. of the certified sick were sent back to work. Of course such an experience is not due solely to improper or careless certification.

Past experience of private mutual sickness insurance societies has doubtless emphasised the fears of the French medical profession as to the new Insurance Law. In this respect the experience of Great Britain is being repeated.

Hitherto it has not been found practicable in France to secure friendly and satisfactory relations between sickness insurance societies and the medical syndicates. The societies have grown in importance, and have usually proved to be stronger than the medical syndicates negotiating with them.

It is urged logically that a free choice of doctors excludes the adoption of any limiting contract, even with the consent of the medical syndicates; but this will not convince the onlookers that it is impossible to make a practical compromise between logic and fairness.

No regulations are laid down in the new French Insurance Act as to the method of paying doctors. It is left to each caisse to negotiate with the medical syndicates as to whether the insured will pay their chosen doctor personally, or whether the caisse itself—the "tiers-payant"—shall pay in accordance with an agreed tariff. As the proportion of the money contributed by the insured which can be allotted to medical charges (15 per cent. to 20 per cent.) is stated in the Act, it will be possible to arrange for personal payments to each doctor; but this will involve enormous clerical work, and there will probably be a balance remaining to be paid by the patient to his doctor. Many disputes will doubtless arise in the settlement of these difficult points.

The medical profession in France are wedded to the conception of "des honoraires payés a l'acte médical", direct payment according to work done; and I may recall that this is the usual system in L'Assistance Publique in France. They object strongly to the speculative element involved in medical work, carried out on contract lines, as, for instance, in England, and with which it may be added English doctors have good reason to be satisfied.

The general proposition that social insurance for medical treatment on a contract basis is degrading to the doctor, lowering his morale as well as that of his patient, will be better discussed in the light of German experience and that of other countries.

In July 1930, at a meeting of the Confederation of the Medical Syndicates, it was agreed by a majority of 8 to 1 to collaborate with the authorities in carrying out the provisions of the insurance law—this decision to be subject to revision should necessity arise.

NOTES ON VISITS TO SPECIAL COMMUNES

The preceding pages deal with the general position in France, so far as it can be judged by interviews with officials and social workers in Paris and elsewhere, and by perusal of available reports and dossiers, especially those placed at my disposal by the Office National d'Hygiéne Sociale.

The description which has been given is necessarily a mere sketch, even for the part of the field of hygienic activities which is mentioned, and the sketch is incomplete. It is intended only to cover the branches of work in which the question of relation between the private and public practice of medicine arises. From this point of view it may now be supplemented by some notes of visits made to special local centres of work.

The Demonstration of the Commune de Vanves.—Accompanied by Dr. Humbert, of the League of Red Cross Societies, I visited Vanves, where I was courteously received by Dr. Lafosse, the enthusiastic and persuasive chief of the work. Vanves is a town of some 20,000 inhabitants, a few miles out of Paris; and here has been formed the Centre de Médicine preventive de Vanves. This has been made possible by a charitable bequest which provides most of the funds. Dr. Lafosse gives his services gratuitously to the commune, as do also his staff. The commune entrusts to him its public health work, and has no other officers engaged in the practice of preventive medicine.

The centre is under the chairmanship of Dr. Roux, the director of the Pasteur Institute, and it is affiliated to the Ecole de Pratique sanitaire de l'Institut Lannelongue d'Hygiène sociale of Paris, whose chairman is Senator Strauss.

The objects of the centre are two: (1) To serve as a demonstration of what can be done in the practice of personal hygiene and the prevention of communicable diseases; and (2) to serve as a field of work or workshop for the Ecole de Pratique Sanitaire, in which can be trained the personnel for public health work.

Dr. Lafosse, in describing his work, emphasised the fact that Public Health is not popular in France; that even when infectious diseases occur, compulsory measures are vexatious, and that consequently the health officer is not always on good terms with the local practitioner. At Vanves success has been achieved in avoiding these stumbling-blocks; and Dr. Lafosse quotes with approval the "marching orders" of Dr. Roux—to proceed "with the good will of the people and the local practitioners".

The chief means to this end has been the use of sanitary nurses (infirmières) specially trained in the prophylaxis of infectious diseases (infirmières sanitaires); but in order to bring these sanitary nurses into favourable relation with the doctors and the people, their services were placed at the disposal of local doctors for nursing their patients (bedside nursing). Their services are rendered gratuitously. There are no other nurses for the sick poor in Vanves, and this lack appears to be fairly general in small communities in France. Their good work in this direction having become appreciated, the infirmières sanitaires of Vanves are now admitted willingly to houses for the prophylactic measures called for in various communicable diseases, including house disinfection, and arranging for vaccination against small-pox, and anti-diphtheria vaccination. Dr. Lafosse lays special stress on this polyvalency of the nurses as a means of securing medical and family co-operation; and there can be no doubt that his tactics are excellent in the present stage of sanitary development of Vanves, and probably also of many other parts of France.

Only four new pupils are taken by Dr. Lafosse each year, these helping the nurses of the institute. There is no formal instruction by lectures, but practical teaching in detailed work.

Special stress is laid on anti-diphtheria work, vaccination with the anatoxine of Ramon being adopted. No cases of diphtheria have occurred in Vanves for several years, though this disease has prevailed in surrounding districts.

Excellent work is being done at Vanves, largely owing to the enthusiasm and devotion of Dr. Lafosse and his staff. Certain reflections necessarily arise from this visit. One cannot but feel astonished that, apart from the devoted work now being done, Vanves should be destitute of the possibilities of elementary sanitary administration; and that there should be no organised arrangement for nursing the sick poor among 20,000 people. And this within an hour's drive of the centre of Paris! The commencement of sanitary work by means of polyvalent nurses is a stroke of wisdom on the part of Dr. Lafosse, and their employment should lead to rapid advance in preventive medicine generally.

Public Health Work in the Département of Aisne.—In visiting the relatively advanced public health work of this département, I had the advantage of the guidance of Dr. G. H. Strode, Assistant Director of the International Health Division of the Rockefeller Foundation, and of Dr. R. Taylor, who is in charge of their work in France and in certain other parts of Europe. Through this co-operation I was able to confer with the Prefét of the Département of the Aisne, and with M. Jean Gullon, Inspecteur Départemental de l'Assistance Publique. We were accompanied also in our numerous visits by Dr. Maurice Chapuis, Docteur de Service d'Hygiène of the Département. To all of these, and especially to Dr. Chapuis, I wish to express my thanks for valuable help.

Starting by automobile from Paris at 8 a.m., we reached Soissons, about 120 miles north-east of Paris, about noon. This town of some 20,000 inhabitants comes within the general range of the public health administration of the département, but it has developed some special local medical services manned chiefly by physicians who are also in private practice.

Soissons was almost destroyed during the war. It is now almost completely a new town, with good housing and excellent environmental conditions. Its public health administration during the war was greatly aided by the Ann Morgan (American) fund, and this remains as a bequest in aid of local public health nursing. These nurses, seven in number, also receive subventions from the State and from private funds. They do all the home visiting (polyvalent) for the town, which, as we have seen, is polyvalent, including the nursing of the sick. The last-named work is stated not to interfere materially with their public health utility. They assist at the clinics and in the medical inspection of schools.

School medical inspection is undertaken by private practitioners, to each of whom is allotted one or more schools. Dr. Bonnefant, the energetic and enthusiastic head of the medical consultations and school medical examinations at Soissons, assured me that but little friction was caused by the examination at school of other doctors' patients. Exceptionally, but rarely, some resentment may have been caused by the suggestion of treatment from one doctor to another doctor's patients. Change of doctors àt school clinics is not permitted by the mayor of the commune at less intervals than six months. Dr. Bonnefant expresses confidence that a fairly uniform standard of school medical inspection is obtained. As a means to this end, he has arranged a change of schools inspected by each doctor, so that, at the end of six years, all school children have been examined by each of the school doctors.

When scholars need treatment, they are referred to their own doctor or to the hospital. No treatment is carried out by the public authority except for teeth. Once a week a dentist attends at a special consultation, and all children without distinction can receive dental treatment gratuitously.

There are three chief municipal consultations in Soissons :—

Prenatal Consultations,
Infant Consultations, and
Dental Consultations.

These are attended by local practitioners.

The Goutte de Lait at Soissons, at which Consultations

des Nourissons are held, is well organised on ordinary lines. Some prenatal consultations are held here. Last year they numbered sixty-three. Only a few cases are sent by private physicians; most come because of the certification required for paying pregnant women to leave off work and for the prime d'allaitement (p. 52). In some départements these payments are made conditional on attendance at the consultation.

Gratuitous treatment of the indigent sick is on the same lines as in France generally. It is arranged from the mayor's office, where prior application must be made, and each case is inquired into.

Soissons has a general hospital of 280 beds, serving also surrounding districts. The hospital has two resident mid-wives (sage-femmes) and thirty maternity beds. Nearly half the births of Soissons occur in the hospital. The usual charge for maternity cases is 20 francs (124 French francs = £1) a day, but some may be charged only 10 francs, and a large proportion are treated gratuitously. Here, as in France generally, the conditions for gratuitous attendance in parturition are much more generous than in respect to disease. Each mother is examined before parturition by the hospital doctor, who decides whether the patient shall be attended by one of the midwives.

Payment for other hospital patients is proportioned to means.

Attached to the hospital is *Le Dispensaire de Sociale Hygiène*, where cases of cancer, tuberculosis, and venereal disease are treated. The organisation of "social hygiene", including in many communities also infant consultations, is separate from that for public health (see p. 54), though through the person of the health officer the two are brought into intimate relation with each other.

At the dispensary the work is done by two of the local physicians. It is not part of the municipal organisation. There is no obligatory notification of cases of tuberculosis; and home visits are seldom made except for patients attending the dispensary.

At the venereal disease division of the dispensary all comers are treated gratuitously, and the facilities for treatment have brought to light many unsuspected cases of syphilis. This work began through the discovery at the prenatal and infant consultations that one-third of the pregnant women gave a positive Wassermann reaction.

Last year 460 births occurred in Soissons. Thirty-eight of these infants died in the first year, 19 of syphilis.

The treatment in a single dispensary of several "social diseases" is worthy of note, as avoiding unnecessary labelling of patients.

The medical administration of the social hygiene work at Soissons by private physicians, so far as I could ascertain, is carried out with little or no friction. Dr. Bonnefant is president of the Association d'Hygiène de l'Aisne (which inherits the residue of the Ann Morgan fund), and he is the moving local spirit in social hygiene.

I next visited Laon, the capital of Aisne, which has a population of about 12,000. The whole Département of the Aisne has a population of about 490,000. Dr. Chapuis is its highly efficient health officer or director of public health; he has a staff of entirely whole-time officials as follows:—

> 5 assistant medical officers,
> 1 laboratory pathologist,
> 40 nurses (infirmières-visiteuses),
> 5 sanitary inspectors.

Automobiles are supplied for the doctors and nurses, and in this direction and in others the International Health Board of the Rockefeller Foundation is giving financial support.

Dr. Chapuis has well-marked and precise views as to the relation of medical practitioners to public health work, which are realised in the distribution of public health medical work in the département.

Thus school medical inspection is done entirely by the assistant medical officers, and private doctors are stated not to object to intimations of defects sent to them. At first Dr. Chapuis attempted to employ private practitioners as school medical inspectors, but with entirely unsatisfactory results for the following reasons. The private physician usually is not a practical hygienist; jealousy was apt to arise between him and other physicians; he often was unable to keep his scholastic engagements; and, lastly, there were no adequate means for controlling varying standards of medical accuracy in inspection. It is found that the present whole-time service costs less, is more efficient, and creates less friction than work by part-time physicians.

But Dr. Chapuis favours using the private physician as far as practicable, especially for work which he can do in his own consulting-room.

Thus, for prenatal consultations, it was found that women did not like to go to the dispensary. They are now sent to a private doctor of their own choice, the département paying for three examinations, at the rate of 10 francs each, at suitable intervals. All women whose husbands do not pay income tax can have this boon. This applies to 75 per cent. of the population. The weak point in the arrangement appears to me to be that the woman must apply first at the mairie for the necessary endorsements. I understand, however, that this weighs but little with the French peasant or workman's wife, because of the collateral financial advantages given by French law (p. 52).

To the infant consultations about one-third of the infants born in the département are brought. Each commune can receive help from the département for the establishment of a consultation, given a minimum standard of attendance.

General practitioners are employed at these dispensaries throughout the département and paid for their services. Where several doctors live in the same commune, a rotation of not less than one year is sometimes allowed, but usually arrangements can be made for one doctor to act indefinitely. For tuberculosis dispensaries, Dr. Chapuis strongly deprecates the appointment of general practitioners. In this instance a greater armament is required, and special skill is needed. The nurses throughout the département are polyvalent. Midwives have attended the majority of births in the past, but now the tendency is to increasing employment of doctors. This was pointed out to me also in Paris and appears to have a psychological basis, the mothers regarding medical attendance in childbirth as a measure of social prestige. Improving means now allow them to satisfy this pride.

I visited also l'Ecole de Plein Air de Lisse, a residential preventorium. Here 170 boys and girls, aged 5–13, are kept for at least six months, being admitted, as the result of medical school inspection or otherwise, with suspicion of tuberculosis or from tuberculous families. About one in ten contribute to the cost of their maintenance. Each child has its blood tested on admission, and 10 per cent. have been found to show a positive Wassermann.

As in other parts of France, the head of the administration is the préfet, appointed by the Government and more or less permanent. The Director of Assistance Publique, M. Gullon, and Dr. Chapuis, Director of Public Health, act directly under him. The préfet practically controls administration, but funds for necessary work have to be voted by the Conseil Général of the Département. There is also an Advisory Commission Générale. In addition, there is a departmental Commission of Social Hygiene, appointed by the préfet, which controls the sale of stamps for tuberculosis and some funds derived from the Government for the social diseases.

Next day I visited Tergnier, where has been built a model garden city, with a population of about 6,000, for railway workers. It is admirably laid out, and comprises sixty-seven types of houses suitable for varying needs.

At Moy-de-l'Aisne I visited a model *health centre* which has been provided by a beneficent lady of wealth. Every need for the treatment of different diseases and for hygienic consultations is provided in consulting-rooms of almost sumptuous character. The district to be served is scattered, and the institution has only recently been opened. The centre is expected to be used by the private practitioners in the district, and the objects of the institution may be gathered from the following summary of its prospective work:—

> It is a centre for outfits for mothers and infants.
> It gives a service of social assistance.
> It loans articles needed for the sick.

It has the following consultations:—

> Prenatal, 1st and 3rd Saturdays at 9 a.m.
> Infants, 1st and 3rd Wednesdays at 9 a.m.
> General Medicine, Tuesdays, 9 a.m. and 8.30 p.m.
> Gynæcology, 2nd and 4th Saturdays at 9 a.m.
> Nose, Throat and Ears, 1st and 3rd Thursdays at 9 a.m.
> Eyes, 2nd and 4th Thursdays at 9 a.m.
> Dentist, 2nd and 4th Thursdays at 9 a.m.
> Radiography, by appointment.
> Surgery, in cases of extreme urgency.

The nurses arrange for home visiting in the communes served by this health centre. The development of the health centre, as a means for bringing about increased unity of action from the clinical and the preventive side of medicine, will be watched with interest.

Public Health Work in the Département of Hérault.—As the result of two days' conferences with Dr. Aublant, the very able Directeur des services d'Hygiène de l'Hérault, and on the basis of the official forms and circulars placed at my disposal, I am able to give a fairly full statement of the progressive health work which has been initiated in this département.

The département is largely agricultural, being concerned chiefly in viniculture. Its people are said to be well-to-do, each small proprietor of a vineyard being prosperous. Their representatives cannot be said to show evidence of this in the parsimonious salaries allotted to their officials who carry on the public duties of the département. School teachers are paid about 100 French francs a week, and the salaries of the six whole-time "médecins-inspecteurs d'hygiène," who are on Dr. Aublant's staff, vary from 22,000 to 30,000 francs per annum, with an addition for

each of 15,000 francs for the cost of telephone, automobile, etc. The highest of these salaries is only about £240.

The present public health organisation dates from 1908,
when the office of departmental health officer was created
by the Conseil Général. Little was done until after the war,
when a subvention of 70,000 francs was made by the
Rockefeller Foundation; and in 1921 plans were prepared
for organising the service, appointing six medical inspectors,
each having charge under Dr. Aublant of a section of the
département. These came on duty at the beginning of 1922.
Since then rapid development of the centralised service has
occurred, as may be seen, for instance, by the following
figures as to the thirteen tuberculosis dispensaries which
have been organised. These are conducted by three whole-
time specialised physicians.

	1922	1927
Number of consultations	599	1,222
Number attending consultations	7,165	17,360
Cases registered (new, first year) ..	2,882	4,780
Home visits	7,347	22,847
Families under supervision ..	1,240	4,086
Sputum examinations	2,224	2,866

That there is much uphill work still to be done is evident
from Dr. Aublant's *Annual Report*. The département has
a population of 500,575. Its birth-rate in 1927 was 14·6,
its death-rate 17·3, per 1,000 of population. Its infant
mortality in the same year was 91 per 1,000 births, and its
death-rate from tuberculosis 1·66 per 1,000 of population.
Its death-rate from typhoid fever was 0·76 per 1,000 of
population.

For several years L'Hérault and neighbouring départements have suffered severely from undulant fever, and
Dr. Aublant and other investigators have demonstrated
that this serious epidemic disease is not conveyed solely
by goats' milk, but that in these areas the sheep is an equal
or even greater reservoir of infection. Thus not only milk
and cheese are responsible for its spread, but also the urine
of sheep, which may contaminate the rural water supplies
from shallow wells. Direct human infection also needs to

be remembered. Present legal powers are inadequate for the control of this disease; and, in view of the general ignorance of the rural population, even the enforcement of existing law is extremely difficult.

The backward position as regards sanitary education is further indicated by the fact that, of the total deaths (663) under one year in 1927, the number returned as due to gastro-enteritis was 216. The work in infant consultations, and more widely in home visits, which is most needed is that of inculcation of elementary precautions in infantile feeding and a higher general standard of domestic cleanliness.

School Medical Inspections.—Each of the six medical inspectors of the département undertakes every section of public health medical work in his own subdivision. Medical inspection of schools and scholars is gradually extending, and already much good work has been done. In 1928, of an effective school population of 26,145, over 23,000 were medically examined, and a beginning has been made in securing treatment of children found defective. A notice is sent to the parent when any defect is discovered, recommending resort to a doctor chosen by the parent. A dossier (carnet) is kept respecting each child examined, and this will be utilised in recommending after-school occupations. No treatment is done by the public authorities, except by the Public Assistance for the poor. Dental treatment is an exception to this. At a municipal school dental dispensary in Montpellier children are treated gratuitously (extractions, stoppings, scaling), but no replacements are made. This arrangement has been approved by the dental syndicalist organisation. The dentist is paid by the city municipal authorities, the lady dentist in charge having been nominated by the dental syndicate, with the proviso that she should not be permitted to engage in private practice.

Dr. Aublant's *Annual Report* is divided into two sections: first, Public Health—the functioning of the services for the protection of the public health; and, second, Social Hygiene—the functioning of the Departmental Office of

Social Hygiene. This subdivision follows naturally from the legislation noted on p. 69. Happily, in L'Hérault Dr. Aublant is largely responsible for the administration of both these divisions of work. In many départements, unfortunately, administration and control are divided.

The constitution of the Office Départemental d'Hygiène Sociale of L'Hérault may be gathered from the following statement. Its intent is to secure collaboration of all local efforts, voluntary and official, concerned especially with the struggle against tuberculosis, and the thirteen dispensaries which have been opened are controlled by it.

The Conseil Général of the département delegates its powers to this office, which consists of members designated by the Conseil and elected for three years. They form a Conseil d'Administration, which then elects an executive committee, for the supervision of the social work coming under the following heads:—

> Specialist physicians,
> Visiteuses d'hygiène (diplomated),
> Dispensaries,
> Specialised hospital services,
> Sanatoria,
> A central laboratory,
> Disinfection,
> Committees for succour,
> Organisation for child welfare.

In each locality L'Office d'Hygiène is represented by a voluntary worker, who supervises local administration. The doctors in each section of work are appointed by the members of L'Office, under conditions laid down by the préfet of the département.

The dispensary doctors, of whom there are three, are required to devote their whole time to this work, including consultations, laboratory, radioscopic and laryngeal examinations. They do not treat patients. The Faculty of Medicine of the University of Montpellier nominates a delegate to inspect the work of the dispensaries, who becomes the technical Councillor of the Dispensaries and a consultant for the dispensary doctors. He is an honorary officer.

Public health nurses (infirmières-visiteuses) are attached to the dispensaries, who also visit patients at home. There are twenty-seven of these and one supervisor. During 1927 the number of families thus under home surveillance was 3,531, and the number of home visits 16,245. These nurses receive salaries varying from 9,250 to 12,050 francs a year, with allowances for expenses in addition. They are forbidden to give any therapeutic advice, but must confine themselves to ascertaining evil home conditions, the needs of patients, and to emphasising the medical advice already given.

For *venereal diseases* an interesting scheme has been devised, which I think will not cover the needs of the community, though it is too early to write dogmatically. Syphilis is a great scourge at present. The scheme for its control is based on an earnest attempt to secure the full co-operation of the entire medical profession. The circular, dated April 9, 1927, introducing the scheme to the notice of private doctors is signed by—

Professor Delmas, President of the Federation of Medical Syndicates of L'Hérault;
Professor Margarot, Chief of the Service of Syphilis and Skin Diseases in the University Medical School; and
Dr. Aublant, Director of the Public Health Services of L'Hérault.

In this circular the difficulty is faced that many patients commonly would not go to their own doctors, and that the doctors not infrequently did not give expert treatment in syphilis and gonorrhœa. It is then stated that more treatment of venereal diseases would be secured if patients could be aided to go to the private cabinet of the physician of their choice. Doctors are then asked to join the new proposed service, the object of which is to place gratuitously at the disposition of the doctor the remedies prescribed by him.

The regulations laid down for patients who elect to go to a private doctor, instead of coming to the dispensary, are intended to extend non-dispensary benefits to all patients capable of conveying infection, to pregnant syphilic women, and to infants with congenital syphilis. Two categories of patients are distinguished: those already on the official list for gratuitous medical assistance, and those who, in the opinion of the selected doctor, should be aided by gratuitous medicaments.

In the first instance the doctor is paid for his work in the usual way for A.P.[1]; in the second instance by the patient.

The gratuitous provision of special drugs is further safeguarded. Each doctor is furnished with special forms divided into three sections. He retains one section, forwarding the two other sections, having entered on the middle one the name of the patient and particulars as to his condition, including the treatment proposed. This is sent marked confidential to Professor Margarot, of the Faculty of Medicine of Montpellier, who, if he approves, forwards the outer third of the form, which is anonymous, to Dr. Aublant, the health officer. Thus the consultant doctor receives a named notification, but not the health officer. From the medical officer's office the medicament is at once forwarded. It is supplied gratuitously to the département from the Ministry of Health.

When a serological examination is required, the specimen, along with the name of the patient, is sent to the Central Laboratory of the Bouisson-Bertrand Institute, which returns a report.

When the information sent to Professor Margarot is incomplete, he can require supplementary information from the doctor in charge of the patient before authorising the issue of medicaments.

The scheme is, as already said, a whole-hearted attempt to secure general medical co-operation in the control of venereal diseases, and it has been approved by the medical

[1] A.P. = Gratuitous Public Assistance.

syndicates. It may be properly stated that the limitations to the supply of drugs appear to be excessive, that it is a pity to limit the gratuitous examination of pathological specimens to doctors adhering to the scheme, and that either free—and fully advertised—access to the dispensaries should be encouraged more actively, or doctors should be specially paid for the entire treatment of patients not regarded as within the range of A.P., subject to their treatment in each case being approved by Professor Margarot as a consultant. Doubtless there will be further developments. Already the principle that in venereal diseases treatment is the chief means of prophylaxis and must be gratuitous has been accepted for dispensary patients, who are treated gratuitously without restriction.

There has been a beginning of visitation by nurses to the homes of patients attending the three venereal disease clinics. This is not regarded as a breach of the confidential character of treatment. The nurses get into touch with patients at the dispensary, and succeed in obtaining invitations to make domiciliary visits. The polyvalency of the public health nurses facilitates this, for the nurses may have to pay visits in a given home in respect of infant care and of tuberculosis, as well as of venereal disease.

Montpellier is the chief city in L'Hérault, with a population of 90,000. It has the second oldest medical school in France, with a large medical faculty, which should make possible rapid improvement in the health conditions of the population of L'Hérault. This end the organisation under Dr. Aublant will attain if adequate monetary support is given, and if a rapid improvement in the hygienic education of the people is achieved. This education at present is evidently at a low ebb.

In the district of St. Francois in Montpellier an intensive effort is being made to demonstrate the possibility of early improvement, which has been supported for several years largely by Rockefeller funds. It comprises the activities already described in a higher degree, as well as educational activities.

This description of medico-hygienic circumstances in L'Hérault would be incomplete without further remarks on the closer co-operation which is being sought between the "functionnaires" of the Public Health Office and the practising doctors in the département.

The position can be seen by reading the following semi-official document:—

AGREEMENT BETWEEN THE DEPARTMENTAL OFFICE OF SOCIAL HYGIENE AND THE FEDERATION OF MEDICAL SYNDICATES OF HERAULT FOR THE WORKING OF ANTI-TUBERCULOSIS DISPENSARIES.

The Federation of Medical Syndicates of Hérault and the Departmental Office of Social Hygiene realise the necessity for collaboration between practising physicians and the physicians of anti-tuberculosis dispensaries.

The Federation of Medical Syndicates does not enter into discussion of the administrative organisation and medical management of the dispensaries of Hérault, which have been approved by the National Committee of Defence against Tuberculosis.

The Executive Committee of the Office of Social Hygiene includes two representatives of the Medical Syndicates, designated by the Federation.

Medical Rôle of Dispensaries.—The aim of the dispensaries, from the medical point of view, consists solely in tracing and reducing tuberculosis. No treatment is to be carried out of any kind under any pretence whatsoever.

The dispensary physicians give prophylactic advice, the carrying out of which at the patient's home is effected under the supervision of hygienic "visiteuses" in concert with the doctor in charge of the case.

The nurse must not arrange to place patients in hospitals, sanatoria, or preventoriums unknown to the doctor in charge.

Dispensary Doctors.—The dispensary physicians are appointed after conference: a delegate of the Medical Syndicate takes part in the appointing committee.

The dispensary physicians ought not to have a clientele of the patients of the dispensary, nor to visit in their homes.

Recruiting of Patients.—As regards diagnosis, any patient presenting himself at the dispensary may be admitted for examination. The dispensary physician should at once advise, by letter, the physician in charge of the patient (own doctor, or doctor of the Bureau de Bienfaisance).

Any patient found to be ill and in need of treatment, and not having his own doctor, is invited to select one from the list of doctors in the area served by the dispensary.

The doctor in charge of the patient, who has been notified by letter from the dispensary physician, should reply, giving all information useful from a medical or social point of view.

After the diagnosis has been established, the patients inscribed will be watched and followed up by the dispensary, except in cases in which the doctor in charge objects.

Once tuberculosis has been diagnosed, especially when tubercle bacilli have been found in the sputum, the patient should be entrusted to the private doctor, and should only attend, at long intervals, at the dispensary consultations. Such patients remain, from a social point of view, under the care of the dispensary, through the intermediary of the home visitor from the dispensary.

Before proposing to a patient that he be admitted into a sanatorium or preventorium, the dispensary physician communicates by letter with the doctor in charge, the latter being asked to give his opinion as to such admission.

Hygienic Visitors.—The home visitors may only enter the families of patients whose names are inscribed in the dispensary when authorised to do so by the dispensary doctor, and after the doctor in charge has been notified.

They should not concern themselves with the treatment of the patients, and thus replace the doctor in charge.

They must not bring any patient to the dispensary without sending preliminary notice to the doctor in charge.

Doctors in charge of tuberculous patients should accept the collaboration of the hygienic visitors in patients' homes and should facilitate their social rôle.

Publicity.—In the waiting-rooms and consultation rooms, the patients should be informed, by notices, of the conditions for admission to consultations.

Patients should equally be informed, by notices, that no treatment is given at the dispensary, and that they ought, in their own interests, to see their family doctor, or go to the Bureau de Bienfaisance for whatever concerns treatment.

The restrictive conditions set out in this document can scarcely conduce to continued efficient treatment of tuberculous patients; and this being so, there is a correlative restriction of hygienic precautions. It may be argued that all the poor can receive treatment through the A.P., but even for them the adequacy of treatment is open to question; and for persons just above the border-line of destitution the severe restrictions on treatment otherwise than by the private doctor cannot be regarded as in the communal interest.

Further remarks on the medical syndicates in France will be found on p. 85.

Public Health Work in the Département of Saône-et-Loire.— Although my visit to Dr. Barrelle, the Inspecteur départemental d'Hygiène of Saône-et-Loire, at his headquarters at Macon, was brief, I was able as the result of my consultation with him, helped by the official documents quoted below, to form a clear idea of the rapid improvement in the health position of the département under Dr. Barrelle's skilful leadership. The departmental health organisation has only existed since the war, and post-bellum developments have undoubtedly been facilitated and hastened by an annual subsidy from the Rockefeller Foundation over a five-year period, which is now coming to an end. The work is actively inaugurated, although incomplete, and there is little fear of relapse into inertia.

The Département of Saône-et-Loire has a population of 549,240. It is divided into 4 arrondissements, 51 cantons, and 589 communes.

As in other parts of France, progress is hampered, and cannot be adequately measured owing to deficiencies in vital statistics. Arising probably out of the exaggerated view commonly entertained as to le secret médical (see also p. 86), certification of causes of death is extremely unsatisfactory, and the local machinery for collecting data and tabulating them is pitifully defective. It is even worse with statements of prevalence of infectious diseases, the notification of which is nominally obligatory. They are belated or entirely lacking in a large proportion of cases; there remains a strong sentiment in the minds of many physicians that such notification is the duty of the head of the implicated household.—In other countries, as is well known, attempts to impose dual responsibility on doctor and the family of the patient have been nugatory, as might have been foreseen on general grounds.—In France, owing to imperfect notification, control of epidemics is difficult and necessarily imperfect.

In Saône-et-Loire the statistical position is stated by Dr. Barrelle to be unsatisfactory. The figures can only be trusted as giving rough indications; and in his report for 1926 he described these figures as somewhat fantastic, while the figures of cases of infectious disease are only a remote reflection of reality.

Subject to the above reflections, the following rates are given, with reservations, in Dr. Barrelle's report for 1928. Death-rate 17·1, birth-rate 16·9 per 1,000 of population; infant mortality, 76·4 per 1,000 births; death-rate from tuberculosis, 1·41 per 1,000 of population.

It will only be necessary to state a few outstanding features of public health work in this département.

The work in puericulture is described as yet in its embryonic stage; but several public health nurses are already employed, and some consultations are held in not very satisfactory quarters. Dr. Barrelle regards the approaching opening of one polyvalent dispensary—which will be concerned with puericulture, with tuberculosis, and with syphilis—as marking a new period in the development of social hygiene.

There are five whole-time medical inspectors on the public health staff, and in 511 out of 589 communes some beginning has been made in medical inspection of schools.

There are five anti-tuberculosis dispensaries at work; and during 1928 6,559 sick persons attended these consultations; 8,841 visits were made at the patients' homes; 1,617 laboratory examinations were made, and 4,789 radiographic examinations; 227 sick were placed in sanatoria and 143 in preventoria.

The chief interest of the position in this département—from the standpoint of the relation between private and public medicine—consists, however, in the arrangements for the prophylaxis of venereal disease by their treatment.

There are five anti-venereal dispensaries, at which, during 1928, 344 new cases of syphilis and 97 of gonorrhœa came under observation. The number of consultations was 17,462, serological examinations numbered 955, and 7,452 injections given (bismuth, mercury, arsenobenzol). Evidently the work accomplished can only relate to a small fraction of the total number of patients needing such treatment. This is fully recognised; and in 1927 was initiated a movement to secure an anti-venereal rural service in the consulting-room of each doctor in the district. In the following statement the regulations for this rural service are summarised. It has been pressed on the attention of the mayor of each commune in a circular by the préfet, the need for maximum publicity being urged. Dr. Barrelle also sent a letter to each practising doctor describing the conditions of the new service and inviting co-operation.

The regulations are based on a letter from the Minister of Health giving his general approval to such rural services, and undertaking to supply the necessary special drugs. They are similar in most respects to those in some other départements, as in Seine-Inférieure, Aisne, Nievre. It is first set out that the new service is intended particularly for venereal patients living remote from dispensaries and who do not come within the scope of A.M.G. (Assistance Médicale Gratuite) as not being indigent, but for whom the cost of adequate treatment is too onerous for their limited resources. Where a dispensary exists, the treatment of such patients should be given in it.

The private doctor who formally enters into this service is instructed to enter on a special "carnet" the following particulars:—

The name of the patient, whether indigent (A.M.G.) or deficient in means (the doctor being the judge);
Result of examination;
Character of injections practised;
Character of drugs used and dose;
Examination of blood, etc.

The same particulars, omitting the name and address of the patient, are to be entered on a detachable coupon, which is sent to Dr. Barrelle monthly. The payment for treatment (apart from gratuitous supply of drugs) for A.M.G. patients is in accordance with the usual tariff for such patients; the payment for treatment of the second class—who may be described as semi-indigent—must be made by the patients themselves.

If consultations are indicated with the expert at one of the anti-venereal dispensaries, e.g. for a serological or ultra-microscopic examination, the préfet can on requisition allow the travelling expenses of the patient.

The arrangements for distribution of requisitioned drugs have been placed in the hands of the General Association of Pharmaceutical Syndicates of France, which designates a local pharmacist as distributor—another instance of special action through the combination representing the interest concerned.

The patient chooses the pharmacist to whom he will apply to make up his prescription.

The control of the new anti-venereal service is entrusted to a technical commission, consisting of the health officer, Dr. Barrelle, and a physician designated by the Federation of Medical Syndicates of the département. They have the right of access to the carnets of a doctor concerning whom inquiry is indicated.

The expenses of the service are borne partly by a subvention from the Minister of Health, Assistance, and Social Insurance, and in part by a special départemental budget.

Somewhat similar criticisms apply to this scheme as to the scheme for L'Hérault. The treatment of venereal disease is hemmed in by formalities and conditions which must limit application for treatment and its continuance, and to the same extent must inhibit the prophylaxis which is the chief object of the treatment. Relaxation of conditions will doubtless occur; and with this and with a greatly increased programme of propaganda and education a great reduction of this scourge—a main cause of premature mortality and sickness—will be secured.

Incidentally the preceding data throw much light on the relation between private and public medicine in Saône-et-Loire. It has been difficult to secure even partial collaboration. When medical inspection of schools was initiated, practising physicians wished to undertake it; the préfet refused to accept the terms proposed for this. The result has been difficulty in arranging for "following up" children who need medical treatment. Dr. Barrelle, in his *Annual Report*, has urged the need for school clinics, at which defects of eyesight, skin and throat conditions, which are usually neglected, can be treated.

Until two or three years ago there was much friction between the A.M.G. and medical practitioners. After much discussion, the older system of a special doctor in each commune for the indigent was abandoned, and the free choice of doctor sanctioned. Now relations are improved. The medical syndicates are powerful, but they do not represent the entire practising profession, and public medical practice as a means for avoiding neglect of disease and consequent disabilities or spread of disease to others happily is growing.

It only remains to remark on the dual public health organisation found in Saône-et-Loire, as in many other départements of France. This arises from the creation of departmental offices of social hygiene, which will eventually need to be completely unified with general public health administration. Dr. Barrelle's *Annual Report* contains a separate section written by M. Pinnette, the president of the Departmental Office of Social Hygiene. The anomaly probably has arisen from the anxiety to develop official arrangements for promoting health alongside voluntary organisations, and with this object all must sympathise.

CHAPTER III

ITALY[1]

PRELIMINARY SUMMARY

The general medical organisation of Italy is not very different from that of France. There is gratuitous medical provision in each commune for the sick poor. So far obligatory sickness insurance is limited to one disease, and this has only recently begun. There is, in addition, considerable voluntary sickness insurance.

School medical work in some centres, as in Milan, is very advanced, and much valuable social medical work for other diseases is also being done.

The organisation of the Italian medical profession on fascist lines presents special features.

GOVERNMENT

The Kingdom of Italy was proclaimed in 1861, and the national system of government then adopted was that of Sardinia, which resembles somewhat closely that of France. In both France and Italy local self-government is restricted by the Central Government to an extent which cannot be said to favour the development of local initiative and patriotism.

Italy is divided into 94 *provinces*, and these into *communes*, of which there are 7,900. The population of communes varies from under 500 to over 1,000,000 (Naples). Each has an equal, and an equally limited, power of self-government. Subdivisions of communes are known as Fractions (Frazioni). The commune is the basis of administrative organisation of the realm.

The *Communal Council* (Consiglio Communale) consists of 15–80 members, according to the size of the place. These are elected for four years. The council elects a mayor (sindaco), who becomes a Government official. It elects also a Municipal Committee (Giunta Municipale) for four years, consisting of 2–10 members, to which supplemen-

[1] Date of investigation, April 1929.

tary members may be added. This giunta is responsible for administration, day by day, including the care of the poor, medical aid, and sanitation.

The communes in combination form *provinces*, which since the Great War have increased from 69 to 94. The prefect (prefetto) of each province is appointed by the Minister of the Interior. He represents the Central Government, and is responsible for public order through the police force; and he has considerable control over the *provincial council* (which is elected for four years) and over the communal councils. He not only controls the legality of the action of the local bodies, but can initiate action and require the local bodies to vote on definite subjects.

The provincial council, like the communal council, elects a *provincial deputation* (now *consulti provinciali*) of 6–8 members, who carry on the executive work of the council, including the care of the destitute and insane, provision of laboratories, etc.

There is, further, a *Provincial Administrative Board* (Giunta Provinciale Administrativa), consisting of the prefect, an accountant, two permanent officials appointed by the Central Government, and five members appointed by the provincial council. This body acts as an Administrative Court, and exercises some control over the activities of local authorities.

The central organ of public health government is the Ministry of the Interior. In this Department is a Sanitary Bureau (Divizione Generale di Saintà), with a number of special sub-departments. It has associated with it a consultative sanitary council. The Central Government, through the prefect, holds a tight rein on local government. In the case of the large municipalities a larger measure of locally initiated enterprise exists; and in time—notwithstanding the centralising paternal governmental changes in Italy of recent years—local government will doubtless become a more living and actual entity. It is only thus that the public—which has to vote through its elected councils the money for all needed public work—will be made willing by self-education to pay for "worth-while" reforms to an adequate extent.

Each prefecture has a *provincial medical officer* and a *provincial council of health*. The provincial medical officer is appointed by the Government. Although perhaps security of tenure is increased by this method of appointment, it is desirable that locally elected bodies should appoint their own officers, subject to satisfactory provisos as to competence for their work, and as to the prevention of unfair dismissal. The provincial medical officer is the pivot of the sanitary administration, collaborating constantly with the

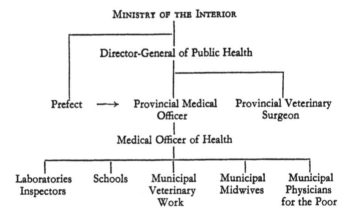

prefect in all technical matters. His general activities are regulated by law. He is required to prepare an annual report on the sanitary condition of the province. This is not published, but is utilised in the preparation of the published report of the Director-General of Public Health for Italy.

In each commune a health officer (*ufficiale sanitario*) is appointed by the prefect on the nomination of the provincial council of health. This health service, except in large towns, is in an infantile stage. In these towns a number of doctors, midwives, etc., are under his control for medical assistance of the poor and hygienic work. The general scheme is shown in the above diagram.

Each commune is under an obligation to pay doctors and

midwives who attend poor persons, whose names have been entered on the communal register of the poor. Under the recent new law of gratuitous medical aid for the poor, several communes of the same province (not more than seven) can combine to appoint a single doctor to attend the poor. This doctor then undertakes in the associated communes the duty of sanitary officer. No similar combination is allowed for midwives. A *Board of Charity* (Congregazione do Carita) must be appointed by the communal council, not more than half of the members of which can be members of this council. They administer the funds of private charities, obtaining their funds from voluntary sources. Since 1870 charitable gifts to religious organisations are subject to the control of the State.

In every province also there is a *Provincial Charity Commission* (Commisione Provinciale di Beneficenza), of which the prefect is chairman. Subsidies are given by the official councils to these bodies.[1] Recent changes have occurred, including the establishment of "Podestas" (appointed by the Government) in the place of elected mayors for places with a population under 5,000. This should mean more satisfactory local government for the smaller units. If these units were combined into larger units, and if, instead of central nomination the election of the podesta was made by the local representatives of the people, a reform of permanent value would be secured. It is arguable, however, with some show of reason that the people of Italy are not yet ready for this reform.

The cost of public health work is shared between the State, the provinces, and the communes. The commune bears the cost of the work of the health officer (ufficiale sanitario) and of the official midwife, and all other expenses within the territory of the commune. The province is charged with the expenses of investigations and work in epidemics, which may be ordered by the provincial medical officer, including veterinary work, etc.; while the State pays

[1] For further particulars see G. Montagu Harris's *Local Government in Many Lands*, 1926.

the salary of the provincial medical officer, half that of the veterinary officers, gives subsidies for other local medical work, and for any special work ordered by the Central Government.

The province of Naples forms an exception to the above scheme of public health administration. Its administration is headed by a High Commissioner. Rome itself has a governor at its head.

Before remarking further on medico-hygienic administration in Italy, one may advantageously describe the work seen in the course of visits made to Genoa, Florence, and Milan. To the officials of these towns I am indebted for great courtesy, for their devotion of much time in accompanying me to see clinics, etc., and for furnishing me with documents from which most of the information which follows has been derived.

GENOA

Genoa is distinguished, from the point of view of facile review, by its publication of an annual public health report. This is written by the Director of Public Health of the City, Dr. Mario Ragazzi, who courteously placed at my disposal Dr. Luigi Guano of his staff.

Genoa in 1927 had a population of 619,484, with a death-rate of 13 per 1,000. In 1922 the death-rate was 17·7. Its infant mortality, which in the past has been as high as 317, is now 135 per 1,000 births.

Dr. Ragazzi's work is carried out under the Communal Administration. The work is divided into nine sections, several of which will now be mentioned.

The first is concerned with *Medical Aid*. It regulates the giving of domiciliary medical aid to the poor, including obstetric care and the supply of drugs, the carrying out of vaccination, the school medical service, the treatment of venereal diseases, and the medical confirmation of certified deaths. For these purposes the city is divided into forty-nine districts, in each of which a communal doctor resides, whose duty it is to give free medical attendance to all those whose names have been entered on the municipal register. This is carried out in accordance with the regulations summarised on page 142.

There are also thirty-two midwives who give corresponding aid in obstetric cases. These midwives must live in their zone of work, and must give their services gratuitously to those on the municipal relief list. They must not refuse assistance in other emergency cases. The midwives are required to retire at the age of fifty-five.

Their salaries are 3,500 lire a year, increased by ten annual increments of one-twentieth. They are allowed to take private cases.

The municipal hospital is supported in part by public funds, largely also by charitable donations and by payments made by patients themselves. Each patient is expected to pay what he can. Vaccination throughout Italy is compulsory in the first year after birth, and again at the age of 8 years. It is done at the expense of the State, irrespective of family means.

Vaccination at the age of 8 is done by the *school medical inspectors*, of whom in Genoa there are twelve, giving whole-time service.

Each school doctor has charge of about three thousand scholars, and frequent visits are made to schools, in addition to an annual special examination of the scholars. Every child found to suffer from defect is the subject of a communication to the parents. In 1913–14 there were 4,319 such cases, in 1926–27 the number was 10,404. A chief part of the work of each school nurse is to urge treatment for defective children. Vigilatrici (school nurses) were introduced in 1919. There are now sixteen of them.

In addition, there are eighteen specialists to whom children are referred by the school medical inspectors for confirmation of special defects. These give "ambulatory" treatment to children whose parents are among the registered poor of the municipality. This treatment includes trachoma, epilepsy, mental conditions, etc.

FLORENCE

My visit to Florence was short, and I was unable to make contact with any sanitary official. At the last census Florence had a population of 245,000. No annual report of its public health work is issued; and most of the work, on its medical side, of combating disease is undertaken by private medical practitioners and by voluntary anti-tuberculosis and similar organisations, and especially by the Italian Red Cross. The chief exception is the organisation for medical treatment of the poor, whose names are on the local register of destitute, which is similar to that in other parts of Italy.

Through the courtesy of Colonel G. Moriondo, Secretary of the Committee of the Italian Red Cross, I was able to visit a tuberculosis dispensary (Dispensaire Antituberculaire Bazzanti) and a preventorium organised by the Red Cross. The tuberculosis dispensary visited by me was admirably arranged, including a radiographic outfit and laboratory. It receives a subvention from the city council, which forms only a small fraction of its total expense. The subvention is limited, as in other communes, to the prophylactic work done by the dispensary. The work regarded as prophylactic includes special aids in diagnosis and visits at the patient's home by the vigilatrici.

Treatment is given to the destitute, including in some instances patients with pneumothorax and tuberculin-treated patients.

The Preventorium ("Anna Torrigiani") was beautifully situated in an old villa of the Medici family in the outskirts of Florence. In this are received some ninety children between the ages of 4 and 10, mostly from families in which there is an open case of tuberculosis. They remain in the institution as a rule until the source of domestic infection has disappeared. This institution was opened nearly two years ago. The arrangements are excellent. It is supported by various voluntary organisations, receiving also a subsidy from the municipality.

MILAN

Milan is a centre of great interest, not only from its varied and almost feverishly active industrial and commercial life, but also because in some respects this city has been a pioneer in progressive medico-hygienic work.

At the beginning of 1928 its population was 927,000, of whom some 56 per cent. are engaged in industry and 12 per cent. in commerce. Of the total industrial population about 24 per cent. are engaged in metallurgical and mechanical industries and an equal number in textile work. Three-fourths of the population of Milan live in tenement dwellings of one to three rooms. The general death-rate has declined from 32·8 per 1,000 in 1878 to 12·5 in 1927. It is difficult to give accurately the death-rate from tuberculosis since large numbers of consumptives die in institutions outside Milan, and there is no complete system of corrected distribution of deaths. But in the year 1926,[1] in which correction was made, the crude total tuberculosis death-rate was 14·42 per 10,000 population; it became 21·52 after this correction. In 1896–1900, without correction, it was 21·62. The need for anti-tuberculosis work is urgent, and it is evident that, notwithstanding the active anti-tuberculosis work already being undertaken, it will be some years before Milan can stand on an equality with cities farther north and west than France.

Two factors in particular impressed themselves on me. In every public building, including public health offices, are provided—e.g. on each staircase and landing—receptacles containing some powder, with a request that spitting except into them should be avoided. The persistence of these, and of the need for them, is a valuable index of sanitary education.

Next I was impressed with the fact—as also in France— that anæmic, rachitic, and undersized children were far too commonly met. And this in a land blessed by glorious

[1] Contribution on *La Lutte contre la Tuberculose* to the Rome Congress, September 1928.

sunshine and a climate encouraging the open life. The character of the tenements, necessitating overcrowding, doubtless counteracts the beneficent work of Nature. So also does the scarcity of domestic fuel, all coal having to be imported. This doubtless discourages open windows and ventilation.

But it appeared to me that a most potent influence counteracting progress both in child hygiene and against tuberculosis, both in France and in Italy, was the inordinate value attached to wine in the national dietary. This doubtless arises out of the fact that the culture of the grape and its manufacture into wine forms a chief industry of the two countries. But the result is no less evil because it has a vinicultural origin. Both children and adults drink too much wine, and children especially drink too little milk. Malnutrition is the chief enemy of progress in health of the young. The preventoria and open-air schools, the helio-therapeutic institutions named in later paragraphs, are doing excellent work; but they can never compensate, except very partially, for the effects of malnutrition in infancy and in childhood, and of the crowded conditions of town life, which might be more rapidly reduced if much expenditure were diverted from wine to milk, from spirits to payment for better and ampler housing.

Doubtless the Italian system of insurance against tuberculosis recently initiated (page 139) will help greatly in hastening the needed reforms.

The progressive medico-hygienic work of Milan is best illustrated in its care of infants, in its school medical work, and in its anti-tuberculosis activities. To view the official and voluntary work in these respects—selected by me—every facility was given through the courtesy of Dr. G. Tron, the head of the Municipal Service for Infectious Diseases, who, in the absence of Dr. Scarpellini, the head of the entire Municipal Department of Health, made all arrangements for me.

Dr. Gutierrez conducted me to the Consultorio Lattanti conducted by Professor Aldo Spalliggi, at the Public Assistance Offices, where valuable work, both prenatal and for nursing mothers, was being done.

To Dr. A. Albertini, the chief of the school medico-hygienic service, I am especially indebted for enabling me to obtain a valuable survey of the admirable work being done for the school child. The information which follows is derived from these visits and from a brochure by Dr. Albertini on the arrangements for pedagogic hygiene of the municipality of Milan. In school hygiene work Milan has been a pioneer in Italy. Its activities include not only all the private and public schools, but also crèches and colonies for climatic cure (mountain or sea).

There are 14 whole-time school doctors, with 44 vigila-trici (school nurses). The work has to cover the needs of about 65,000 children in 90 primary schools, of 5,000 younger children in municipal and an equal number in private crèches, as well as of 15,000 pupils in other schools and colleges.

The various schedules employed in investigation are not reproduced here, but they are unusually complete and elaborate, and it is patent that the work is well done. I can only summarise this most briefly. Each doctor takes charge of a certain number of schools. Each of these schools is visited weekly, the doctor remaining at the school from nine to twelve and two to four o'clock. Every school has a special room for the doctor. New scholars are made the subject of a complete examination, and a general examination is made of every child twice a year. Each communal crèche is visited weekly by the doctor. Each scholar is revaccinated at the age of 8 years. Small ailments are attended at the school by the doctor or by the school nurse, who is always present with the doctor. School nurses visit each school three or four times a week.

I visited a large school, "Caterina da Siena", which has some 1,400 pupils of all ages from the crèche upwards to 14. The building was perfect for its purposes; but I was assured that other schools in Milan were as good. The classes were not too large; only two scholars were allowed for each desk. The arrangements for drill and gymnastics, including class singing as part of the gymnastic training, were admirable.

But the most impressive portion of the school was its educational crèche, where six young children—infants and children of 2 or 3 years—are brought daily by their industrially employed mothers and kept under model conditions. Girls in the eighth class, aged 13–14, take their turn, under supervision, in tending these infants, preparing their food, and keeping them clean, washing the clothes, etc. Every girl is passed through this instruction. There is a similar crèche in another part of Milan.

As is too well known, a large part of the medico-hygienic work of school doctors consists in the discovery of already established disease, and in securing its treatment.

At the beginning of the school year 1926–27 the number of new scholars who were examined was 9,601, and of these the percentage suffering from skin affection was 2·3, from phthisis nearly 1 per cent., from open tuberculosis of glands or bone over 1 per cent., from naso-pharyngeal obstruction 14·2 per cent., from cardiac affections 1·8 per cent., from visual defects 4·4 per cent., etc.; 21·1 per cent. were suffering from general weakness.

The arrangements for treating any malady which is detected consist in referring the parent of the child either to the private doctor of the family or, failing this, to the public assistance. There is, in addition, a special service for treatment, the school polyclinic.

School Polyclinics

School doctors refer special cases for consultation, and sometimes for treatment, to the specialists of the school polyclinics. These number eighteen and are open daily. All important specialities concerned in child health are included. The specialists give their diagnostic services gratuitously for all school children without distinction, but treatment is undertaken only for those children whose families are entered on the municipal list of indigents. The extent of consultative and curative work undertaken at these polyclinics is seen from the following table for 1928 :—

	Brought for Consultation	Treated
Pediatrics	265	113
Internal medicine	226	240
Ophthalmic	1,060	230
Ears, nose, and throat	1,326	646
Dermatology	423	232
Radio-therapy	33	29
Neurology	52	24
Radiology	500	—
Anti-tuberculosis dispensaries .	2,860	648
Pedagogic medicine	232	180

Dental treatment of children is undertaken once a week at each school by the Stomatologic Institute acting on behalf of the municipality. Mobile dental cabinets are provided for this purpose.

There is no evidence of conflict or friction in the arrangements between private doctors and the school doctors. There is little scope for this owing to the meagre wages which prevail and the inability of a large part of the population to pay for medical care. There are said to be more doctors than the community needs, and their earnings are small. Notwithstanding the excellent medical work which is being done, it cannot be said that the standard of earnings either of physicians or of the patients treated by them is at all satisfactory.

A labourer earns 25 lire (about 5·4 shillings, or 1¼ dollars) a day. A doctor seldom gets more than 10 lire a visit. The communal doctors for the poor receive 800, or perhaps 1,000, lire a year. They may have, but are said not to obtain much, private practice in addition.

On the large scale much medico-hygienic treatment of school children is undertaken.

I was conducted over the open-air school "Umberto

di Savoia" by Dr. C. G. Cristina, of the Municipal Tuberculosis Service, and conferred also with Signor Leone Clerle, its director. This school receives two classes of scholars: some 1,500 children who come daily and have their dinner at the school; and some 200 other specially selected children who reside in the admirably arranged residential part of the school and remain there sometimes for the entire duration of school life, 6–14. The arrangements for meals, for douche-baths, for swimming, for sunbaths, for gymnastic and general instruction were admirable. Pupils are admitted on the recommendation of the school doctor from among tuberculous families or because of specially feeble physical condition. The educative gymnastics, including choir singing, were well graduated; and in every department personal hygiene was taught.

At this school there is also a summer open-air school for 2,500 children.

There can be no doubt that in these schools, as well as in the summer colonies (sea and mountain) which cared for some 20,000 children in the summer of 1927, much good is being done beyond the immediate personal good secured. They promise for the next generation a wide appreciation of hygiene and a rapid decrease in tuberculosis and nutritional diseases.

Milan opened the first school in Italy for mentally defective children; and the work done in this "Z. Trèves" school under the direction of Dr. Albertini is important. It is carried on entirely at the cost of the municipality. There are seventy pupils aged 6–14 years. Each of these is personally studied, a complete dossier of his heredity, previous circumstances, present condition and progress being kept. Furthermore, two visiting nurses are continuously engaged in following up ex-pupils, and in helping them in various ways. Without this, as Dr. Albertini states, much of the value of the carefully graduated school training would be lost. Use is made of the medical pedagogic "ambulatoire", which visits the school weekly in order to give expert help for special conditions.

The work, as in most communities throughout the civilised world, is only at its beginning. Seventy pupils are received; but the number of mentally defective children in Milan probably is ten times this number. Elaborate investigations in such schools should throw light on causation; and in illustration some figures relating to the work in this school may be quoted. Though scanty in number, they point to one direction—the prevention of syphilis—for much reduction of feeble-mindedness.

I give only the grouped figures, which comprised altogether 313 children suffering from mental defect, neuropathic lesions, or epilepsy. In these several groups the proportion which gave a positive Wassermann test for syphilis varied from 72 to 86 per cent.; a proportion which assumes significance when it is stated that of the children in open-air schools in Milan only 10 to 12 per cent. gave the same positive reaction.

Tuberculosis Service.—Tuberculosis work in Milan, as in other parts of Italy, is partly official, but chiefly of a voluntary character. The State and the commune grant subsidies to approved agencies; each province has propaganda in common, the provincial anti-tuberculosis associations and the Italian Red Cross being active in this field.

The various anti-tuberculosis measures of Milan and the province are centred around *prophylactic dispensaries*, which have increased in Milan to six since the year 1912, when the first communal dispensary was opened. The work of these dispensaries remains difficult, owing to deficiencies in means for meeting the fiscal needs of consumptives and their families.

As in France, the principle is adopted that the municipal dispensaries shall be exclusively prophylactic in function. The dispensary is a centre of investigation and of hygienic advice, including domiciliary counsel. Already it is noted that these investigations have been the means of analysing the circumstances of some 42,000 Milanese families.

The six dispensaries are distributed in different zones of Milan. Four of them are municipal, and two are closely associated with the municipality, but are conducted by the Institute of Phthisiology and the Milanese Association against Tuberculosis. The personnel of these six dispensaries comprises 12 doctors, 12 tuberculosis nurses, and 10 other employees. They are open every day, including Sunday, but excluding Friday, which is selected for the weekly rest.[1] Each dispensary is provided with a laboratory and X-ray apparatus. When consultations are required, the municipal consultants (page 137) are available.

Most of the home visits to dispensary patients are made by the nurses; but on the nurse's first visit she is accompanied by a doctor, who thus becomes personally acquainted with the social circumstances of his patient. In these visits only prophylactic work is done, and thus any reason for frigidity between the "family doctor for tuberculosis", as he is named, and the private doctor who treats the patient, is said to be avoided. Evidently these relations call for the utmost tact. For patients who cannot afford a private doctor the communal doctors for the poor become in practice doctors attached to the dispensary.

Specialised ambulatory assistance is given by means of three "ambulatoires". They are intended chiefly for patients who have already had special treatment in various institutions, and for whom its continuance is indicated.

Hospital or sanatorium treatment follows dispensary diagnosis in a considerable proportion of cases: and Dr. Guizzon is emphatically of opinion that, in the circumstances of the Milanese, home treatment should be avoided. "Hospitalise to the greatest possible extent, and for as long a time as possible." Also this should be done with the minimum of bureaucratic restrictions.

I am indebted to Dr. C. G. Cristina for demonstrating the extremely important work being done in one of the dispensaries under his charge. Some six thousand patients attend this dispensary in the course of a year; and it is evident that really high-class work is being effected.

An expression of admiration of the work done in Milan

[1] See Dr. Guizzon's contribution to *La Lutte contre la Tuberculose.*

for nurselings, for school children, and for consumptives is called for. It is extremely promising, besides being already fruitful in results. Perhaps what is most needed, in addition to an extension of present work, is a continuous educational campaign directed to improved hygienic habits of the people. The work to this end in the schools must in time be most effective; and it may be that much more work than I know of is being done in education of parents and other adults in the important part which personal and domestic hygiene plays in citizenship.

To this end the new law enforcing

OBLIGATORY ASSURANCE AGAINST TUBERCULOSIS,

which came into operation in May 1928, should give an important impetus.

With the possible exception of syphilis, against which efforts of control are being developed, there is no preventible disease so threatening to the public weal of Italy as tuberculosis.

The following are the chief conditions of this assurance and of the insurance against invalidity and old age which preceded it. It is easy to forecast that compulsory invalidity insurance, and now special compulsory insurance against tuberculosis, will be followed by more general insurance for sickness when the financial conditions of Italy permit of the extension.

Insurance against Invalidity and Old Age.—By a decree of December 30, 1923, insurance against invalidity and old age was made obligatory for males and females aged 15–65 who are employed by others. This includes industrial workers, labourers, shop-assistants, and all employed in domestic science, in industry, commerce, agriculture, public works, etc. It does not, however, apply to those whose wages exceed 800 lire a month (92.5 lire = £1), to sailors employed on the ships of other nations, to agents and employees of State railways, etc., for whom special schemes exist.

The scheme provides aid in the prevention and cure of

invalidity, pensions for old age, and for those permanently incapacitated, and certain payments in the event of death.

The contributions to secure these benefits for the insured are as follows:—

	Paid Fortnightly (Lire) by the	
	Employed	Employer
If daily wages are less than 2 lire ..	$\frac{1}{2}$	$\frac{1}{2}$
If daily wages are 2–4 lire	1	1
If daily wages are 4–6 lire	$1\frac{1}{2}$	$1\frac{1}{2}$
If daily wages are 6–8 lire	2	2
If daily wages are 8–10 lire	$2\frac{1}{2}$	$2\frac{1}{2}$
If daily wages are over 10 lire ..	3	3

Contributions are usually made by fortnightly stamps on the personal cards of the insured, the employer being responsible for affixing these.

The benefits commence at the age of 65, subject to certain conditions. They are proportionate to the contributions; they include payments to the widow and children under 15.

The administrative arrangements are in the hands of the National Office for Social Insurance (Instituti di Providenza Sociale). There is a Council of Administration, including an equal number of representatives of the employers and employed, as well as officials of Government departments.

Institutes of Social Providence are formed in every province, except when several provinces combine for this purpose. These are subordinate to the Central Institute. They undertake local supervision and individual payments.

Insurance against Tuberculosis.—By a national decree dated May 20, 1928, it was enacted that in view of the urgent need to institute insurance against tuberculosis this should be enforced on a compulsory basis for all persons of both sexes who are insured against invalidity and old age under the decree of December 1923.

Tuberculosis being one of the chief causes of premature

invalidity and of the production of widows and dependent
children, the need for such insurance—as a means of
avoiding excessive burdens on the invalidity insurance
funds—is fairly evident, though it is secondary in importance to hygienic measures.

Under this Act the Ministry of the Interior is empowered
to arrange for the necessary machinery. The aims of insurance are to provide for insured persons and their families
special places for treatment of tuberculosis, including sanatoria and post-sanatorium homes, and to ensure separate
institutional treatment in recognised hospitals under satisfactory sanitary conditions.

The family of the insured under the Act includes husband
or wife, legal and natural children, and brothers and sisters,
not over 15 years old, who are living in the same house or
at the charge of the insured person. Servants in the house
have the same rights.

The benefits accrue after not less than twelve fortnightly
contributions during the two years previous to application.
The contributions fortnightly payable in lire to ensure
these benefits are from the—

	Employed	Employer
Daily wages up to 8 lire (1 lira = 3.50 pence)	$\frac{1}{2}$	$\frac{1}{2}$
Daily wages beyond 8 lire	1	1

Similar arrangements to those for invalidity insurance
apply for tuberculosis insurance. When assistance is required,
this is given after investigation by the anti-tuberculosis
association of the province. An appeal lies against refusal
to help by provision of treatment or financial aid. The
insured person with dependents has the right to a daily
allowance for his family, which is proportional to the
contributions paid by him in the previous six months.
This amounts in the higher class to 4 lire, and in the lower
class to 6 lire, a day.

If institutional treatment is given, part of the benefit is
apportioned for this. When no beds are available, home
treatment is accorded, with a daily money allowance.

The details of organisation of help are worked through the Cassa Nazionale per le Assicurazioni Sociali acting in co-operation with each Consorzi provinciali anti-tubercolari.

For further particulars see *Casta del Lavoro*, Art. XXVII, commented on by G. Bottai, Under-Secretary.

MEDICAL ATTENDANCE ON THE POOR

District medical officers are appointed for each commune, as indicated on page 128. Their duties may be gathered from the following summary of the regulations for this service (*Capitolato per il Servizio Medico*, 1925) which determine the work of medical attendance on the poor in Milan. These may be taken as fairly representative of corresponding rules in other parts of Italy.

The stipend of the district doctors is not controlled solely by the number of poor persons inscribed on the official list for his district, though this number serves as a basis on which the stipend is established.

The list of poor persons is revised annually, and the district doctor is expected to assist in this revision.

Additions to the list may be made during a year; but they only take effect—except for emergencies—after a month.

The district doctors are appointed by the communal council, on the strength of their qualifications or by examination, or both.

The appointment is made at first for two years, and the doctor during this period is subject to three months' notice. If then reappointed, he is not subject to removal.

The condition is made that vacancies shall be made known to the various medical organisations.

The doctor appointed must have been three years in practice and be not over 35 years old. Unless otherwise arranged, he must live in his zone of work, if possible centrally. Over his door must be placed the words "Medico Municipale", and he must be in direct telephonic communication with the pharmacist of his district. He must call thrice daily at this pharmacist's address to ascertain any "calls".

The hours for calls are subject to regulations. Inattention to calls is subject to disciplinary action.

In cases of difficult labour the district doctor must render help to the district midwife; and he can arrange for institutional treatment when necessary in such cases.

When sent for at night, the doctor can demand to be accompanied by the person fetching him out and back.

The doctor must undertake minor operations. For more serious cases he can require consultations and help.

He must whenever practicable treat his patients at their homes, and only send them to hospital when lack of assistance or the nature of the illness makes this necessary. Official inquiries are needed before hospital treatment is given.

In the event of disaster or in any emergency the district doctor must give his services, even though the patient is not on his official list or lives in another zone.

Each day he must have definite consultation hours at a centre provided, where there is also a nurse.

He must give free medical certificates as required, including those needed for school or occupational attendance.

He is required to keep a register of visits and consultations and send a copy to the health department.

It is part of his duty to make autopsies and report on his findings as required; and to give all necessary death certificates in cases in which an autopsy is not needed.

He is required to supervise the midwives in his district and infants who have been entrusted to wet-nurses.

In infectious diseases he must assist the health department when required.

He has the general duty of supervising the general hygiene of his zone, and especially of the dwellings visited by him, and of reporting on these to the health department. He is required to give a short report on this subject at the end of each year.

He is required to vaccinate gratuitously the inhabitants of his district, and must control the results of vaccination, and supply certificates.

In prescribing drugs he is required generally to adhere to an authorised list of drugs.

There are special rules as to absence from work and deputies.

His salary is 8,500 lire a year (92.5 lire = £1), subject to ten yearly increments of one-twentieth of his salary. An additional 500 lire is given if the poor in his zone number more than 1,200.

He is provided with free travelling in the municipal tramcars.

It will be seen that the district medical officer is in reality a combination of a poor law medical officer and a medical officer of health, an arrangement identical with that holding good in most sanitary districts in England in its earlier public history from 1860 to 1880 or 1890. The combination was abandoned in England for reasons which are given elsewhere (in a concluding volume), but there is much to be said for it so long as the interests of private practice are not allowed to interfere with adequate care of the poor and the wider health duties.

THE ORGANISATION OF ITALIAN DOCTORS IN SYNDICATES

Although, as seen in the preceding pages, public health authorities have undertaken but little treatment of disease, and medical obligatory insurance is limited to invalidity and to one disease (tuberculosis), there now exists a carefully conceived and executed professional organisation of the medical profession which has a definite bearing on our main problem.

The Fascist revolution has been followed by the organisation of doctors in a new combination of Corporate Syndicates for the carrying out of important duties. These duties comprise the giving of assistance and counsel in matters of hygiene, with a view to the improved health and greater productivity of the workers of the realm. The medical syndicates are also intended to promote scientific study and to protect the conditions of professional work.

In accordance with this duality of objects, which are convergent, there are "professional orders" and syndicates, which are complementary in function.

The professional orders keep the medical registers of qualified doctors, and guard the discipline and decorum of the medical profession, in relation to its members and to the general public and sick persons.

Prior to Fascism the professional orders settled disputes between doctors and their clients as to the payment of fees. Now this task is left to the medical syndicates. These syndicates fix professional fees, examine disputes as to these, and frame the advice on which magistrates decide in cases in which there are legal disputes. The medical syndicates are largely represented in the council of the professional orders, and thus have a voice in determining their policy. In this way they have a moral as well as an economic task; they bind together the scientific medical societies and aid them in developing their activities.

The Italian medical syndicates are unlike corresponding organisations in other countries, for they have a political character, being profoundly Fascist.

All doctors who are inscribed in the National Fascist Party belong to these syndicates; other doctors are admitted who wish loyally to collaborate in securing the social and political objects of the régime.

Doctors outside the syndicates are entitled similarly to be inscribed in the registers of the professional orders, if they are legally entitled to practise medicine in Italy.

Medical officials of the State and of communes are grouped in separate associations and are forbidden to develop any syndical activity. The Fascist conception means, in effect, that the sovereign right of the State would be infringed to a certain extent if the State's officials were syndical, and that there was thereby implied the idea of a bi-lateral compact of work. The State in substitution gives its officials a juridical position, and provides for them a special defensive organisation. Any official differences are settled after a judicial hearing. But as very many medical officials are also engaged in private practice, they resume their right to be included in a Fascist syndicate, in matters solely concerning them in this latter capacity.

The medical syndicate undertakes the making of agreements with private institutions, with insurance societies, with private houses of health, and with factories and other institutions which utilise medical services for themselves or for their employees. The contracts of work thus made enter into precise detail as to salaries, hours of work, terms of employment, and invalidity and old-age insurance.

In Italy there is no obligatory insurance against all diseases; but many mutual societies and employers have voluntary systems of sickness insurance. For these many contracts have already been settled, and others are in train. These guarantee the conditions named above; they also define the maximum number of insured to whom each doctor can give medical aid, so that overcrowding of patients may be avoided and an adequate number of doctors may be employed.

The medical syndicate protects economically not only its own members, but also other doctors in the practice of medicine. The sole privilege of members of the syndicate consists in the fact that they can guide syndical activity, both in relation to current contracts of work and to sanitary legislation.

In the definite judgment of those consulted by me, the new system of organisation of the Italian medical profession has had a powerfully beneficial influence on its economic position, and has aided greatly in drawing the attention of the State authorities to the desires of the profession.

The medical Fascist organisation in each province has a secretary and a director, elected by its members. These provincial syndicates are affiliated to the National Medical Fascist Syndicate, which was founded in 1922. This central organisation, like the provincial, is organically connected with the corresponding syndicate of workers, from which its social and political attitude is largely directed. This union between the two is regarded as fundamentally important.

From the present time it is intended that every contract of work will have as its condition that the worker is insured, so that he may have medical and other aid in illness; this, as it develops, will mean a national system of sickness insurance entrusted to the syndical organisations of workers and their employers.

The previously noted insurance against tuberculosis is an important step in this direction.

The development and working of the above elaborate machinery for control of the medical profession in its relation with its constituent members and with the public will be watched with interest. It is characteristic of a highly developed and centralised organisation in which individual action must bend completely to the will of the community as expressed in the syndicate. If future difficulties arise, they will emerge especially in the relationship between the medical and the workers' syndicates.

Much active *Maternity and Child Welfare Work* is being done in Italy, and especially in efforts to protect children against tuberculosis. It is unnecessary for our purpose to describe the various institutions having this object beyond what has been written under the local headings.

ANTI-ALCOHOLIC WORK

In nearly every European country publicly organised efforts are being made to reduce the damage to health and efficiency caused by the alcoholic habits of a section of their population. Italy is no exception to this statement; and as appears appropriate in a country in which the individual is to be regarded as an instrument for increasing the efficiency of the commonwealth, it is not surprising to find that recent drink legislation in Italy embodies the following points:—

1. Voluntary drunkenness is to be regarded as an aggravation of a crime and not an extenuating circumstance.

2. No kind of alcoholic drink may be sold to children or young people under 18; and

3. Licences for the sale of alcoholic drinks, which at present number 1 to every 200 of the population, are in future to be limited to 1 to 1,000 of the population. Expiring licences will not be renewed until this proportion is reached.

PUBLIC MEDICAL WORK AGAINST PALUDISM

The State and the communes take an active part in the treatment of malaria, as a means for its prevention. Large quantities of quinine are distributed gratuitously or at reduced prices at the cost of the State. The distribution is made by the provincial authorities through local pharmacists.

PUBLIC MEDICAL WORK AGAINST VENEREAL DISEASES

By enactments made in 1923 and extended in 1926, gratuitous treatment of venereal diseases is provided, not only for the indigent, but free dispensaries have also been provided for the entire population. Such dispensaries are obligatory in the chief town of each province and in all towns with a population exceeding 30,000. It is proposed to make the establishment of an anti-venereal dispensary compulsory in every industrial establishment having more than 2,000 workers! The cost of dispensaries is borne by the communes, with the aid of subventions by the State. In 1927 the number of dispensaries aided by the State was 187.[1]

Hospitals are required to treat venereal diseases while contagious at the cost of the State. The State, furthermore, has established anti-venereal dispensaries in sixteen ports at its expense.

[1] See *L'Hygiène Publique en Italie*, Geneva, 1928.

CHAPTER IV

JUGO-SLAVIA[1]

INTRODUCTORY

What follows in the main is a sketch of hygienic conditions of that part of the new Kingdom of the Serbs, Croats, and Slovenes which is called Croatia. (Since October 1929 the new kingdom is to be known as Jugo-Slavia.) Before describing the fruit of my personal observations in and around the capital of Croatia, reference should be made to the recent history of this remarkable new country. The tragic story of Old Serbia in the Great War, including the history of its decimation by typhus fever, is well known. Perhaps not so well known is the great work carried through by the Serbian Child Welfare Association of America. Had it not been for the great financial aid rendered by this and other American agencies, and still more the devoted personal work of its agents in Serbia, the story of that country would have been even darker than it was, and its remarkable recovery and still more remarkable hygienic advance could not have been realised. If I do not describe in full the village centres or zadrugas which have been opened in various villages by voluntary agencies, with the aid indicated above, it is not because the great value of their medical and educational work is not fully realised. Training-schools for nurses have been established by or with the aid of the Serbian Child Welfare Association of America at Belgrade and Valjevo, and thus one of the most urgent needs of Jugo-Slavia, the provision of sick nurses and public health nurses, will gradually be provided.

The health zadrugas have so far had rather a medical than a public health function. This is inevitable, the treatment of disease necessarily having priority over the more general steps needed for its prevention. As elsewhere, it will be found that treatment is a most valuable opening

[1] Date of investigation, May 1929.

not only for personal hygiene, but also for securing the broader work of public health.

The official health work of Jugo-Slavia owes much of its rapid growth and wide scope to its official chief, Dr. A. Stampar.

Dr. A. Stampar is the head of the hygienic section of the Ministry of Health, now become the Ministry of Public Welfare, and his leadership and genius, his personality, and uninterrupted power to influence Parliament in the direction of reform under changing political conditions, and now under temporary autocratic rule (September 1930), have given a great impetus towards the important and in some respects drastic medico-hygienic reforms already secured.

It is likely that the terrible experience of Jugo-Slavia of smallpox, and still more of typhus during the Great War, made the representatives of the people willing abetters and promoters of the reforms now organised. If this be so, Jugo-Slavia has but repeated the experience of Western nations—sometimes "fever", sometimes smallpox, sometimes plague being the provocative agent of reform.

To realise the complexity of the work required one needs to realise the different races and civilisations now included in Jugo-Slavia. These are so diverse in character and in social development that it would not be inapt to think of Jugo-Slavia in this respect as a miniature India.

The effort being made throughout Jugo-Slavia is to bring medical aid and counsel within reach of everyone, and thus render preventive work universally possible. The zadrugas and the increasing provision of nurses—these represent mainly voluntary work, rendered possible by grants in aid from abroad—have been supremely important in this crusade. They are being supplemented by official organisations. The central hygienic institute (one in each of the nine banats or provinces) is described later on. In addition, there are about 80 district health institutes and some 500 village stations. The last-named have, or are intended to have, departments for maternity and child welfare, school

clinics, clinics for tuberculosis and venereal diseases, a
small bacteriological laboratory, a museum, and a bath-
house. The health officer of the district is in charge of
these. Liberal support to this work has been given by the
Rockefeller Foundation.

Evidently this ambitious programme implies frequent
points of contact and of possible conflict with the relatively
few medical practitioners in Jugo-Slavia who are engaged
in private medical work; and it is remarkable that, notwithstanding the incompatibilities of almost impossible parliamentary politics, reform still progresses.

SPECIAL DESCRIPTION OF CROATIA

What follows is in the main a sketch of hygienic conditions of that part of Jugo-Slavia called Croatia. This was
the only part of the most complex new country, the Kingdom
of the Serbs, Croats, and Slovenes, which I was able to visit.

I came to Zagreb by road from Fiume, a distance of
ninety-six miles, travelling, during the greater part of the
ten hours' trip, over mountainous roads in regions with
a sparse population. It would not have taken so long but
for the fact that at the time of my journey (April 26, 1929)
many of the roads still had snow on them, and in others,
specially near several great timber centres, the roads were
indescribably difficult from thick mud, with boulders
irregularly distributed below the mud.

But the journey enabled one to realise the difficulties of
a medical and hygienic service in such regions. The problem
for these mountainous regions is not dissimilar from that
of the Highlands and Islands of Scotland and of some
mountainous regions in Kentucky and North Carolina. In
all of these alike local resources are unequal to the task,
and there is a moral call on central governmental funds,
not yet adequately answered either east or west.

Zagreb itself is an open, pleasant town, with many
wide streets and good architecture. It has a University,
and is the centre of varied and apparently prosperous
activity.

Of the total population of 141 millions in Jugo-Slavia as a whole, 7·7 millions are Roman Catholics, 5·6 millions Greek or Orthodox, 1·3 Muselmans (Mohammedans), while there are smaller number of Jews and Protestants.

The chief industries of the country are rural, and it is a country of small cultivation and of human labour. The spade and the hoe are much more in evidence than the plough in the parts of Jugo-Slavia outside Croatia.

An excellent description of the organisation of the Public Health Services in Jugo-Slavia has been given by Dr. Stampar in one of the publications of the League of Nations. Here it is only necessary to give an outline which will enable the reader to place my account of different branches of medico-hygienic work in their proper setting. It is well to bear in mind that Jugo-Slavia was only formed in December 1918 out of Serbia, Montenegro, and certain countries of the former Austro-Hungarian Empire. The laws and administration in these different parts show marked variations.

In 1918 the new Government was organised into seventeen ministries, each with a cabinet minister at its head, under the King and Parliament. Two of these ministries dealt with Health and Social Politics. These have recently been amalgamated into one ministry.

In what follows I am concerned chiefly with Zagreb, town and country, in which I was able to make personal inquiry. In making this inquiry my path was rendered smooth and easy by the help given and the facilities placed at my disposal by Dr. B. Borcic, the Head of the Hygienic Institute of Zagreb, and Dr. J. Rasuhin, the Head of its Department of Social Medicine.

CENTRAL HYGIENIC INSTITUTE.

On this institute public health administration largely depends for its guidance and control. In each of the *nine hygienic provinces or banats* into which Jugo-Slavia has been divided for public health work, this is even more the case. The almost complete absence of prior local public health administration outside Croatia has rendered possible the new economical and satisfactory administrative arrangements which have been made; and those who belong to countries in which local administration in small and unsatisfactory units is part of their national history may in this respect—I do not say in other medico-hygienic respects—envy Jugo-Slavia in having begun its work without the impedimenta which undue multiplication of units and administration implies.

Jugo-Slavia, for political representation and administration, is divided into thirty-three departments. It is by fusion of these thirty-three that the nine hygienic provinces or banats have been formed.

On its governmental side the Zagreb Central Hygienic Institute is in direct relation with the Hygienic Department at Belgrade, which, under the Minister of Health and Social Politics (more recently the Ministry of Public Welfare), is conducted by Dr. Stampar.

The Central Hygienic Institute is concerned on one side of its activities with investigation and research of public health problems, and on the other side with administrative control of the hygienic province (department) of Zagreb.

This combination of research and administration, in the circumstances of Zagreb, is eminently satisfactory. There is little risk of administration becoming stereotyped and rigid, so long as it is closely linked with scientific investigation of current problems. There might conceivably be risk of the gradual encroachment of the needs of daily administration on the opportunities for research, but this is, I think, satisfactorily avoided by the organic integration of the Central Hygienic Institute with the School of Public Health on the same site. This owes its existence to the Rockefeller Foundation.

THE SCHOOL OF PUBLIC HEALTH

As this school constitutes a fundamentally important part of the public health work of Zagreb, and as its staff also are an essential part of its public health organisation,

I interpose here a short description of the activities of the school. The school is intended as a centre of teaching of every branch of public health, and to aid by giving expert help in all efforts for improving the public health.

Its teachers are University professors or members of the staff of the Hygienic Institute, and the same Director (Dr. Borcic) controls both establishments. He is appointed by the King on the nomination of the Minister of Health and Social Politics. The Advisory Board is thoroughly representative of all medico-hygienic activities. The school is supported in part from State subsidies and other sources.

The school, in combination with the institute, comprises the following divisions of work:—

DEPARTMENTS WITH SECTIONS

1. Of administration.
2. For bacteriology and epidemiology.
3. For biologic products.
4. For chemistry.
    (a) For the analysis of victuals.
5. Anti-rabic.
6. For the production of smallpox vaccine.
7. Hospital for infectious diseases.
8. For parasitology.
    (a) For zoology.
    (b) For phytopathology.
9. Technical.
    (a) For rural sanitation.
    (b) For sanitary engineering.
10. For social medicine.
    (a) For the propaganda of health.
    (b) For the studies of national pathology and for statistics.
    (c) For public instruction.

The closeness of the relation between administration and laboratory work will be seen from the following examples:

The bacteriological-epidemiological department is concerned with the control of local infectious diseases in conjunction with the district health officials, with giving aid in bacteriological and serological diagnosis, and with inspection of subsidiary laboratories, ambulances, disinfecting arrangements in the districts.

The department for biological products supplies all biological preparations for active and passive immunisation to local doctors, besides manufacturing these preparations and investigating their potency. Smallpox vaccine lymph and anti-rabic lymph are manufactured in the fifth and sixth departments of the institute.

There is a hospital abutting on the institute in which cases of acute infectious disease are received for treatment from Zagreb and its vicinity. Patients pay for their maintenance in the hospital, if they can afford it.

The Social Department of the School.—The department of social medicine forms an important part of the institute and school, and I give here the official account of its multiform and valuable activities carried out under the direction of Dr. Rasuhin; for on the application of the principles taught in this department depends largely the health and welfare of the Jugo-Slavia of the future.

(*a*) Expert supervision over all establishments of social medicine on the territory of the institute.

(*b*) Study of social and sanitary legislation.

A. *Section for Hygienic Propaganda*

(*a*) Maintenance and organisation of popular lectures.

(*b*) Publication of books, pamphlets, posters, etc.

(*c*) Preparation of moving pictures and erection of a film studio.

(*d*) Keeping a central library and a special printing plant of the institution.

(*e*) Keeping and arrangement of a museum and organisation of periodical hygienic exhibitions.

B. *Section for the Study of National Pathology and for Statistics*

(*a*) Study of the conditions of life, lodging, and nourishment of peasants and workmen.

(*b*) Discovery of good and rational methods for the improvement of public health.

(*c*) Study of the various diseases among the population and their special etiology.

(*d*) Gathering of statistical information on births, diseases, and mortality of the people.

(*e*) Study of the biologic and anthropologic peculiarities of the people in general and of the different groups.

(*f*) Statistical elaboration of the reports and works of all sections of the institution.

(*g*) Scientific work, lectures, and practical exercises in the laboratories and in the field.

C. *Section for Instruction of the Population*

(*a*) Working out projects and organisation of regular and periodical courses in the institution.

(*b*) Working out scientific projects for all schools for assistants and hospital attendants in the country.

(*c*) Organisation, instruction and control of auxiliary sisters, nurses, laboratory attendants, disinfectors, market inspectors, etc., on the territory of the institute.

(*d*) Organisation and supervision over schools and courses for housekeeping.

(*e*) Control over schools for midwives and organisation of courses.

(*f*) Organisation, instruction, and supervision over the school for physical education, collaboration with and support of all private efforts aiming at the physical education of the population.

(*g*) Co-operation in health and pedagogical work with all other establishments of similar nature in the country, also keeping in touch with such establishments abroad.

(*h*) Providing for expert publications devising new tools and instruments to be used in health pedagogy, also experimental work pertaining to health pedagogy.

As an illustration of the wide spread of the activities of this department may be mentioned a two weeks' course for barbers on the hygiene of their calling.

The school and the institute form the central brain of public health organisation for the hygienic province of Zagreb.

Locally they are linked to the following organisation:—

Homes of public health	3
Public health stations	12
School clinics	16
Infant and child welfare centres ..	7
Treatment centres for venereal disease	15

Treatment centres for trachoma .. 9
Treatment centres for malaria 6
Health centres and sanatoria 3
Public baths 14
Various other institutions 8
Bacteriological epidemiological insti-
tutes 3

FREE MEDICAL TREATMENT OF THE POOR

The Administrative Department of Zagreb is divided into eight districts, and each of these is subdivided into from five to eight *communes*, each with its own elected local governing council. By the national law each commune is required to pay a communal doctor. His duties are to supervise local sanitary administration, to inspect the schools in his sanitary commune, and to undertake any work in forensic medicine that may be required. He must also attend the sick poor gratuitously. He undertakes also private practice; but in some communes few are excepted from the right to gratuitous medical treatment. If a commune cannot afford a "living wage" for a doctor, several political communes in a sanitary commune may combine to employ the same doctor.

The right to gratuitous treatment is based on the fact that the man's taxation by the State does not amount to 10 dinars (about 20 American cents) per annum. If a doctor considers that an applicant for treatment should pay his fees, the patient must obtain a certificate as to his taxation: gratuitous treatment is given without question unless the doctor requires this testimony.

About 80 per cent. of the population are peasants or small farmers, and probably one-third of these do not pay 10 dinars a year in taxation. In each commune there is also a midwife supported in part out of communal funds.

Hospital treatment, when required for those entitled to gratuitous domiciliary treatment, is paid for at the public expense. Others must pay according to their means. In Croatia each of its three political departments has a collective sanitary fund, into which the constituent communes pay 25 per cent. of their local taxation; and the cost of doctors, midwives, and hospital treatment is defrayed from this fund. This fund is controlled by the representative council of the department. Towns and autonomous sanitary communes do not pay into this fund, but make separate arrangements.

I am unable to say whether these arrangements for the treatment of the poor are generally satisfactory or adequate. In view of the poverty of rural communities, the sparseness of the population, and the general circumstances of the country, it is probable that the service needs very extensive supplementation to meet the needs of the people.

Each of the thirty-three departments of Jugo-Slavia has a representative council, the members of which are elected for four years. The council for the department of Zagreb has gone farther than others in providing gratuitous medical treatment. Medical men in this province are paid 5,000 dinars a month (about £220, or $1,000 a year) to treat, without distinction, all applicants who are ill. Each of these official doctors has a definite area allotted to him, but patients apparently need not keep to the doctor in their own area. As the doctor's payment does not depend on the number of patients he receives, this arrangement may be embarrassing to the conscientious doctor, who has become a favourite in virtue of his good professional work. Patients in the province of Zagreb, as elsewhere, have to pay for maintenance in hospital, unless they come within the above-mentioned limit; and this supplies a judicious check (by the patient) on the doctor who wishes unnecessarily to transfer his patient to a hospital.

The Zagreb arrangement has only existed for a year, and it appears likely that it will need to be modified in the light of experience.

It should be added that private medical practice continues in Zagreb. This suggests a close analogy with scholastic experience in England, where general taxation on the entire community supports the communal schools, but a considerable proportion of the parents thus taxed continue to pay large fees and to send their children to schools which do not benefit from general taxation.

The physician of each commune is under the control of a district medical officer (acting for several communes), whose salary is paid by the Central Government. This D.M.O. is appointed by the Government, the local governing bodies having no control over his activities. He is, in fact, the M.O.H. (Medical Officer of Health) for his area, and is responsible for sanitation and the control of epidemics. For public health purposes the physician for the poor is subordinate to him; but if there is no physician for the poor, the district physician must treat them when sick. Both of these officers undertake vaccination, which is compulsory and gratuitous; but the communal council is required to pay half a dinar for the lymph with which each person is vaccinated, the funds from this source going towards the expense of the Hygienic Institute.

In the town of Zagreb much good work is being done for *infants and pre-school children*, though evidently not yet on a scale which is commensurate with needs.

Dr. Svare, the head of the first-class centre at which most of this work is done, showed me each department of his work. There is a prenatal consultation centre conducted by a lady doctor, which meets three times a week. Patients are brought by midwives and public health nurses, sometimes twelve on one day, although the centre has only been open for a few months. Most of the patients are sent by midwives, sometimes as early as the second month of pregnancy.

I may interpolate here that there is a school for training midwives in Zagreb, at which two years' training is required. Established midwives are required every four years to undertake a course of post-graduate training, and they must attend. They are sent by the district medical officers. Midwives engaged in private practice are required also to undertake this training.

MIDWIFERY SERVICE

As already indicated, every commune has its midwife, who attends normal confinements gratuitously for the poor, her income thus being derived chiefly from official sources. A patient requiring a doctor must pay for him, unless the head of the household comes within the scope of free medical treatment.

CHILD WELFARE CENTRE

The centre in Zagreb, which is directed by Dr. Svare, is supported in part by the municipality of Zagreb and in part by the State. As in other departments of social and medical work, voluntary agencies count for little in Jugo-Slavia. Nor is this surprising in view of the extreme poverty of the majority of the people and the low remuneration of the professional classes.

Every midwife is obliged to intimate at once all births occurring under her care; and in Zagreb last year over 93 per cent. of all births were thus notified.

The public health nurse visits the family within the first week after birth; but as there are only four of these nurses for Zagreb, not more than one-half of the families are visited, and revisits are infrequent. In 1927 the rate of infant mortality in Zagreb was 147 per 1,000 births. Many sick babies are brought to the centre by their mothers, and if poor these are treated. Occasionally some objection has been raised by private practitioners; but the ability to pay a private doctor is so exceptional in the class of people who attend the centre that this point rarely arises.

The institution has been at work since 1908, and throughout its career the giving of cows' milk pasteurised and in bottles, each bottle containing enough for only one meal, has formed an important part of the work. The distribution of milk is so managed that it does not, in Dr. Svare's judgment, ever form an inducement to substitute unnecessarily artificial for breast feeding. The municipality owns forty cows, all tuberculin-tested, from which the milk needed for this institution and some hospitals is derived.

The centre has a number of cots in separate glass-protected cubicles for infants needing in-patient treatment.[1] These are treated and isolated on strict Pasteurian principles. Thus it would appear all the dangers so notoriously associated with the hospitalisation of young children are avoided.

An interesting part of the work of the centre is the provision for wet-nursing. By arrangement with the town's obstetric hospital, five mothers recently confined are transferred with their infants to the centre, and there kept for several months. The infants are kept as in-patients, being fed by their mothers, who lodge in a separate part of the centre. The same mothers are utilised for wet-nursing other specially feeble inpatient infants. The mothers themselves do laundry work at the centre until the social workers of the centre are able to arrange for them and their infants to be placed satisfactorily at home or otherwise.

It is found that from 3 to 4 per cent. of the infants coming to the centre have syphilis. Once a week there is a special clinic at the centre for the treatment of this disease, and a similar weekly clinic for tuberculous infants.

In the year some 2,800 infants and children aged 1–4 attend the centre, making some 21,000 visits. I was impressed with the thoroughness of the work done at this centre, and with the methods of ensuring that social help and guidance go hand-in-hand with the highest medical care.

School Medical Service

School Medical Service.—The arrangements for medical care of elementary school children are as follows:—

In rural districts the physician of the commune or the district physician is required to see each child when entering school at the age of 7. Special attention is paid to those with physical or mental defects.

The health inspection of school children in Zagreb is

[1] The use of the word "treatment" does not necessarily imply that the infants are sick. The treatment given may be merely the needed social help.

organised more completely. Zagreb has twenty-two school doctors, specially skilled in children's diseases, also one doctor for ocular conditions and one for dental defects, and eight school nurses. Each child is examined on entering the school and yearly by the doctor and nurse. A dossier is prepared and kept, and the parent is informed of any defects and asked to confer with the doctor. Advice is given for all; treatment for the poor. The children who have defects are seen several times in the year. Nurses attend to parasitic conditions and help in arranging for baths, etc. There are two sanatoria for delicate children, one at the sea, and one in the mountains; and every year some 600 children from the Zagreb schools are sent to them, the selection being made at the school polyclinic.

After the elementary school (7–11 years) comes the middle school (11–19 years), either gymnasium or real school; then the University. At the University a five years' course is required for medical students.

The arrangements for boys and girls in middle schools in Zagreb were of a high order. At these schools adolescents from 11 to 19 years old are taught gratuitously and receive a large amount of medical care. For the elementary school in Zagreb the municipality are responsible. The middle schools are supported by the State, which is thus responsible for the socialisation of medicine—to the extent to which, as seen below, it is carried—as well as for higher education.

I do not reproduce here the complete dossier of the medical activities of the middle school authorities in Zagreb, for which, and for demonstrating the complete system, I am indebted to Dr. Desenka Ristovitch. The headquarters of this school work is at the school polyclinic, at present housed in temporary buildings, to be shortly replaced by more elaborate premises. The work began some four years ago, and already is in full working order. The following points distinguish this service. (1) Each year every student is under an obligation to receive a complete physical examination by a doctor. No exceptions to this are allowed.

(2) Every scholar is eligible for treatment at the polyclinic without any social distinction whatever. This privilege is extended to all University students. The treatment includes dental treatment, correction of eye defects, and of abnormal conditions of nose and throat, as well as more general conditions and tuberculosis. There are spray baths attached to the polyclinics to which all students have access, and the majority of students utilise this privilege weekly. Last year there were some 40,000 attendances at these baths.

Obviously a complete system such as this cannot have been organised entirely without protest, especially on the part of private medical practitioners. Probably owing to the sparsity of doctors, opposition has been almost negligible. The official logic of the situation is that people pay taxes proportional to their social and financial status, and thus the treatment cannot fairly be limited to the poor. When challenged by an individual physician, Dr. Ristovitch debates the point with him in friendly fashion, the burden of her argument being that, until the school doctor found the condition needing medical treatment, it had remained undiscovered or neglected; and that once it was discovered the student or his parents had the choice as to where treatment should be done. In the circumstances of Zagreb —in which there is financial restriction in nearly every class—the State, i.e. the co-operative, method of meeting the problem appears to have been the only one likely to ensure success. Like education, medical treatment for students up to 18 is thus gratuitous.

SCHOOL MEDICAL INSURANCE

A modified system on the basis of insurance will shortly come into operation for the entire country. The scheme for this has already been passed by the State Parliament.

Under this scheme a Students' Fund will be created, out of which the expenses of medical treatment of students will be defrayed. Each student (or his parent) will pay 20 dinars a year, and each student in the University will pay 60 dinars a year, and will thus be insured for any medical care required during his student life, for such treatment as can be given at school clinics, presumably not for any medical attendance that may be required in his own home.

Some protests against this legislation have been made by private doctors, but the overwhelming opinion of the public is in its favour. It forms a remarkable scheme for improving the health of the on-coming generation, the progress of which will be watched with interest. Reference may be made to the Swiss scheme (Vol. I, page 239), which differs, however, from this in providing also domiciliary medical attendance, and in giving treatment not at special clinics, but only by the doctor of the patient's own choice, who works according to a detailed tariff.

TUBERCULOSIS

Tuberculosis is a terrible scourge in Jugo-Slavia. According to the statistics collected by Dr. Stampar (in the League of Nations' publication), which are recognised to be imperfect, it is fairly certain that in Croatia-Slavonia the death-rate from all forms of tuberculosis is considerably over 4 per 1,000 inhabitants. In the town of Zagreb in 1908–18 the recorded death-rate from tuberculosis was 6·5, and in Belgrade in 1900–10 was 8·7 per 1,000 population.

The first reason for this excess that suggests itself is the poverty of the population; but this is only a secondary, not an essential, explanation, for, as Dr. Stampar points out, the tuberculosis mortality is very high among the Serbs and in the Voyvodina, "which is a very rich part of the country." Dr. Stampar places as chief factors, first the lack of sanitation, drink acting as a contributory cause, and then the superstitious concealment of the disease, leading to protracted exposure to infection.

In Zagreb I visited the tuberculosis dispensary under the guidance of its chief, Dr. Vladimir Cepulic, who showed me the details of its valuable scientific and practical work. He is associated in the work of the dispensary with one assistant doctor and four nurses, who help in the work of the dispensary, and also make social inquiries and give hygienic advice in the patients' homes.

During last year 427 new patients were treated at the dispensary. The number of deaths in Zagreb from tuberculosis in the same year was 458.

The dispensary receives notification of open cases of tuberculosis from sickness insurance doctors (1,071 last year), and the Health Department of the municipality notify all deaths certified as having been caused by tuberculosis. Following on these intimations, domestic disinfection and cleansing are carried out, an attempt to examine "contacts" is made, and the public health (tuberculosis) nurses give hygienic advice.

Private doctors send very few patients to the dispensary, and very few specimens of sputum come from them; although in each instance gratuitous help is offered. But in connection with the national insurance scheme (see below) many sputa are received for examination.

It is evident that much uphill work will be necessary before anti-tuberculosis work begins to have the success which eventually is certain. Some additional facts throw light on the present position. In Zagreb 458 deaths from tuberculosis occurred in 1928. Of these 113 occurred in hospitals. Out of 2,300 hospital beds in Zagreb, only 30 are available for tuberculosis.

A complete ledger is kept at the dispensary of the deaths from tuberculosis in every house in Zagreb. In one religious establishment—a monastery—year by year something like 6 per cent. of its inhabitants have died from tuberculosis. After each death disinfection and cleaning of the room occupied by the deceased has been carried out, a very necessary work. But it has not been possible to undertake the systematic examination of all the monks, the surveillance of doubtful cases, the segregation of open cases, etc., without which it is evident that the holocaust may continue indefinitely.

Another important conclusion emerges from the municipal death statistics, as analysed by Dr. Cepulic.

He finds that more than half of the deaths occurred among the relatively well-to-do, who form much less than half of the total population. Evidently, then, poverty is not the essential determinant of excessive tuberculosis in Zagreb. The poor, if of hygienic habits, escape infection; and Dr. Cepulic concludes that it is the class of the "hygienical proletariat"—for the poor include a large proportion of professional and other intelligentsia—which have turned the balance against the well-to-do, who are ignorant and superstitious and persist in habits speading tuberculosis.

In a communication to the *American Review of Tuberculosis*, February 1927, Dr. Cepulic has further emphasised the essential point in the prevention of tuberculosis. He concludes that "we must, once and for all, give up saying that some houses are breeding places for tuberculosis," and must conclude that "tuberculosis is not linked up with houses or flats; it is linked up with foci of disease." Of course this conclusion does not imply that insanitary and overcrowded dwellings have no importance in favouring tuberculosis; but Dr. Cepulic's conclusion, based on experience at Zagreb, is consistent with experience in England and America. Foci of disease must be removed. Failing this, the opportunities for infection *in situ* must be minimised by every hygienic possibility. The position may, not inaptly, be compared with that of a remote country village which had been free from enteric fever for a long series of years, although the inhabitants of this village were supplied with water from shallow wells in the immediate propinquity of foul sanitary conveniences. No obvious disease occurred until (as in William Budd's classical example) a servant girl returns home from a distant town in the early stage of an attack of enteric fever. In the next few weeks almost the entire village was "down" with the same disease.

Hope for the future lies in practical action based on this conception; and the immediate task is one of education of the medical profession and of the general public in the elementary tasks of hygiene.

An instructive, even if ludicrous, illustration of the need for elementary hygiene is that of the use of cuspidors. I do not suggest that dried sputum, subsequently scattered, is the chief or sole means of spreading tuberculosis; but carelessness in this respect is symptomatic of corresponding carelessness in unprotected coughing, in hygienic care of the sick, etc. A poor man attending a public institution was observed to expectorate at intervals on the floor. The nurse each time placed the cuspidor near him, but without succeeding in impressing its object. The poor man finally said to the waiting patient next to him: "If she keeps doing that, I shall be obliged to spit into it!"

Parenthetically, might not the progress of anti-tuberculosis measures be symbolised by a study of the use of cuspidors? First, there are none, and indiscriminate spread of infection occurs. Second, they are provided more or less, but their utilisation is unskilled and imperfect, their cleaning is often neglected, and the provision made may be said to encourage undiscriminating expectoration. Third, in Western countries—some of them—cuspidors have disappeared, and the act of coughing is safeguarded, but there is much less expectoration than in the communities in which they are provided.

The hope of the future is wrapped up in the hygienic instruction of the people, in the visitation of all infected homes by tuberculosis nurses, in the work of the tuberculosis dispensary, and perhaps more than all in the fact that attendance at the tuberculosis dispensary in Zagreb forms an essential part of the work of medical students at the University, with its hopeful forecast of improved ideals in the medical profession generally.

Anti-Alcoholic Work

In Croatia some effort has been made to control alcoholism. By law it is forbidden to sell any alcoholic drinks during the days before and after and on the day of an election for parliament. The tax on saloons and other premises in which alcoholic drinks are sold is double that of other shops; and some educational work against alcohol is officially promoted. This is especially so in all hygienic institutes.

SICKNESS INSURANCE

The system of national sickness insurance to meet the medical needs of scholars and students does not complete the story of social medical insurance in Jugo-Slavia, for there is also a national system of sickness insurance for all employed workers. In its present form this applies to the whole of Jugo-Slavia, having been in force since May 1922.

Before that, various laws for social insurance existed in different parts of the present Jugo-Slavia. In Dalmatia and Slovenia there had been compensation for accidents from 1887 and a Health Insurance Act from 1888. The latter was obligatory. The maximum contribution was 3 per cent. of the wages, two-thirds of which was payable by the employer and one-third by the employee.

In Bosnia and Herzegovina sickness insurance was also obligatory on similar lines. In each instance sickness and maternity benefits were given, as well as monetary payment during twenty weeks of 60 per cent. of the sick person's wages. In Serbia a law dating from 1910 provides for insurance in regard to sickness, accident, old age, and death.

To unify these various laws was a very difficult task, but in 1922 this was accomplished.

Every person who hires himself out for work, whether physical or mental, is bound to be insured, whatever his earnings may be. The wages of unskilled workmen are from 24 to 45 dinars, and of skilled workmen from 45 to 100 dinars a day. Only persons earning less than 40 dinars a working day are exempted; and, in addition, persons otherwise insured, as State employees on railways and miners. Workers not coming within the definition of "employed" can join the scheme voluntarily.

All voluntary schemes are superseded, one national scheme taking their place. The central office for the national scheme is at present in Zagreb; there are twenty-six local offices throughout the Kingdom. The central office is organised in accordance with the national law. There is a general assembly consisting of representatives from the twenty-six local offices, and the assembly elects a board of directors. These select the president and two vice-presidents, who, with the general manager (Milan Glaser), constitute the supreme board. I wish at this stage to express my appreciation of the courtesy of the last-named and of Dr. D. Hahn, who gave me the details incorporated in this report and showed me over the magnificent central insurance building in Zagreb, with its polyclinics and baths.

Members under the national scheme are insured against disease, accidents, and disablement.

So far as disease is concerned, the physicians of the district offices elect from among them the board of health of the central office, which consists of twelve members. This board of health appoints three delegates to the board of directors. The entire national scheme is under the supervision of the Minister of Health and Social Politics.

Provision is made for the settlement of disputes in special courts, consisting of State judges and twenty jurors for each court. Appeals from this court are heard by a Supreme Court, which also consists of judges.

Contributions.—Insured persons are divided into seventeen wage-classes:—

Class   I. Daily remuneration under 2.50 dinars.
             Insured on an average for the daily sum of 2 dinars.

.   .   .   .   .

Class VIII. Daily remuneration 8 to 9.6 dinars.
             Insured on an average for the daily sum of 8 dinars.

.   .   .   .   .

Class XVI. Daily remuneration 34 to 40 dinars.
             Insured on an average for the daily sum of 34 dinars.

.   .   .   .   .

The contributions payable for health insurance amount to 6 per cent. of the daily wage. They must not exceed 7 or be lower than 4 per cent. of the wage. Within these limits they are adjusted to cover all expenses. One-half of the contribution is paid by the employer, and one-half by the employee.

For disablement, old age, and insurance of survivors the contribution must not exceed 3 per cent. of the wages; but this section of the national scheme we need not follow farther. Contributions for insurance against accident are in accordance with a schedule of the particular occupational risks, as officially settled.

The law requires the Government to pay annually one million dinars in aid of disablement insurance, and the same amount for accident insurance.

Benefits.—Under health insurance there is secured in sickness—

1. Medical treatment for twenty-six weeks, including drugs, medical and surgical appliances;
2. Payment for the same period of two-thirds of the insured person's wages.

Furthermore, insured women are entitled to—

3. Medical help and a midwife in parturition; and
4. Three-fourths of the insured woman's wages for two months before and two months after confinement. Special premiums are given to women suckling their own infants, not exceeding 3 dinars daily.

The dependents of insured persons when sick and living in the same house as the insured person are entitled to medical treatment, drugs, and appliances during twenty-six weeks, also medical help and a midwife during parturition, with a maternity benefit of $1\frac{1}{2}$ dinars for one month before and one month after confinement. Dependents do not include collateral relatives.

Survivors of an insured person receive a sum equal to thirty times the daily earnings of the deceased worker.

The national scheme includes some 460,000 members, or about $3\frac{1}{2}$ per cent. of the total population of the Kingdom. If dependents are included the proportion becomes about

6 per cent. This small proportion is an interesting indication
of the small amount of employed labour, the majority of
the population being peasants who live on their own
holdings. These do no come within the scope of the
scheme, except on a voluntary basis; and in 1924 there were
only 2,238 persons in this category.[1]

The weekly contributions are collected by a large staff
of collectors. It has not been considered practicable in the
circumstances of Jugo-Slavia to entrust the employer with
this task. Collection is difficult, and I was informed what
in four-fifths of the cases payment had to be enforced by
legal action, but that, nevertheless, not more than 0·2 to
0·5 per cent. of the amounts owing were lost. These
conditions must imply a heavy percentage cost for administration, which should, however, decrease with time. It is
possible that the collectors may be made useful in health
propaganda; the value of this use of collectors has been
shown in the industrial insurance experience of the Metro-
politan Insurance Life Company of New York. If the same
collectors could be utilised in other local work for public
authorities, further economies might be secured.

The Treatment Given.—About a thousand doctors are
employed in insurance work in Jugo-Slavia.[2] Each doctor
thus employed is elected for the purpose by the insurance
office, the directors of which represent employers and
employees in equal proportions. There is in the strict sense
no free choice of doctors for the insured. Only those
doctors on the official list can be employed, and sometimes
this means in a given area a choice of only one doctor.

The directors of national insurance regard the limitation
of choice of doctors as a great safeguard against abuse of
sickness benefit, and as making it easy to ensure that the

[1] A valuable outline of the National Scheme is given in a brochure by
Dr. Zeljka Hahn, 1925.
[2] For Jugo-Slavia as a whole I cannot give the number of doctors, but in
Croatia, with a population of 2·7 millions, they number 700. Of this number,
86 are in State or communal service and without private practice, 186 are
in private practice only, 300 are in State or communal service and in private
practice, and 77 are in private and insurance practice; some also are in
private practice and also hold appointments under the State and insurance.

interests of the national fund are maintained against undue demands. This is so, although the appointed doctor also has private patients; for the patient cannot change his doctor, except for reasons satisfactory to the local insurance office.

The service of general practitioners is supplemented by ambulatoria in nearly all towns and large industrial centres, of which there are about thirty altogether. The larger ambulatoria have peripatetic specialists, dental departments, X-ray apparatus, and chemical and bacteriological laboratories. Special sanatorium treatment is also provided. The insured patients can select their own consultant.

It is claimed by the insurance chiefs that the present national organisation gives a satisfactory service; while under the old poor-law system treatment often is a "fiction", and is commonly inadequate and unskilled, the supply of doctors for the poor not being equal to the needs of the community. Evidently, although the insurance system represents a great national advance in medical service, it likewise only meets the needs of a relatively small proportion of the entire population. In the town of Zagreb there are only six doctors for the statutory poor among some 130,000 people. Of these one-half are stated to be in the technical sense paupers.

The economic conditions of Jugo-Slavia make medico-hygienic advance very difficult; and in view of this the progress already made is astonishing. To ensure more rapid improvement in health, certain conditions will need to be fulfilled, and realisation of some of these does not appear to be very hopeful at present. It is said that on two subjects the people of Jugo-Slavia are always prepared to spend money—military preparedness and public health. The international position appears unhappily to make continuance of the first form of expenditure inevitable, though the more is the pity! But in certain other directions, as in the consumption of alcoholic drinks, great economies are immediately possible; and it remains always axiomatically true that effective sanitary and medico-hygienic reform, including temperance reform, brought about by educational effort and judicious legislation and administration will almost immediately secure a reduction in the terrible burdens imposed by disease, and will go far towards ameliorating the economic conditions of the country.

CHAPTER V

HUNGARY[1]

PRELIMINARY SUMMARY

Hungary's public health and medical work is seriously handicapped by *postbellum* conditions. In its evolution the State Hygienic Institute and the Institute of Social Hygiene are bearing an important part. Medical remuneration is most inadequate. All wage-earners are compulsorily insured against sickness. The insured do not have free choice of doctor. Polyclinic treatment is highly, perhaps over, developed. Other medico-social activities are described in the following chapter.

My examination of medico-hygienic work in Hungary was rendered pleasant and easy by the active assistance given and by the readiness to confer on all doubtful points shown by a large number of public men, physicians, and hygienists.

To Dr. Cornelius Scholtz, the Secretary of State of Hungary, I am indebted for an interview in which was summarised the information already received. To Dr. Georg Gortvay, of the Social Hygiene Institute, and to Captain Horvath, the secretary of this institute, I am indebted for guidance and help; and to Dr. Gortvay in enabling me to meet in pleasant circumstances a group of experts in medicine and hygiene. I was fortunate in meeting Dr. Leland W. Mitchell, the representative of the Rockefeller Foundation, in whose company and that of Dr. J. Tomesik, in the absence of Professor Johan, its chief, I visited the State Hygienic Institute, for which Hungary is indebted to American munificence. Other names are mentioned in subsequent paragraphs. I was accompanied in most of my visits by Dr. Karl Schubert, a young expert in biometrics, a former student of Johns Hopkins University.

[1] Date of investigations, April–May 1929.

Hungary is full of vitality and energy, though greatly distressed and embarrassed by the consequences of the Great War. In the words of the Secretary of State, "the mutilation of the country by the Trianon Peace Treaty has created a parlous situation also with regard to public hygiene." That, notwithstanding this, there is much public health activity, and especially notable developments in medical insurance, will be seen hereafter.

The population of Hungary is only 36·4 per cent., and its area 28·5 per cent., of the pre-war condition. Not only so, but most of the richest parts of Hungary, especially of mineral wealth, are now in foreign territory. It may be that Hungary is fortunate in one respect: its Army is restricted in numbers by the treaty conditions, whereas those of its neighbours, who have gained territory from it, are spending excessively on war-preparedness, a circumstance which means wastefulness in an undesirable direction, and parsimony in the much-needed expenditure on the health of the people.

GOVERNMENT

The various local authorities—subject to much financial control—have more local autonomy than exists in Latin countries. In the present reduced territory there are 12 municipal and 25 county councils, related centrally to the Hungarian Parliament, to the Government, and to the Regent. Each county and municipality has as its head a prefect (föripan) appointed by the Government, the local authorities in counties electing a vice-president (alispán) and in towns a mayor (biró) as representing the self-governing side of administration. In each county or town there is a municipal committee, one-half consisting of the highest taxpayers and one-half of members elected for six years.[1] In addition, there are administrative and advisory committees, and a special advisory municipal health committee, consisting of experts in equal numbers with representatives of the municipal committee.

[1] See Harris, *Local Government in Many Countries*, p. 161.

In smaller communes there are also councils with a small group of executive officers; and in each commune taxes can be raised by adding centimes to the national land-tax and certain other taxes. In each commune there is a district medical officer, appointed for life. In towns these officers are appointed by the municipal councils.

In Budapest there is a chief burgomaster (lord mayor), elected by the municipal council from three persons nominated by the Head of the State. In each county and town there is a chief medical officer: in Budapest administration is carried on in ten sections, each with its medical officer, and controlled by a councillor. In Budapest these medical officers are appointed for six years by the municipal council; in other areas for life. In addition to the medical officers, there are also communal and town doctors, for treatment of the sick and to help in promoting the health of the community. Each commune with not less than 5,000 inhabitants must employ such a doctor; smaller communes combine for this purpose. These doctors give gratuitous treatment to the poor, but can charge those not in this category according to a scale fixed by the local council. Usually the fee fixed is from 2 to 3 pengös per patient (4 pengös is about equivalent to three shillings in English money). They also undertake vaccinations (which are obligatory), certify deaths,[1] and control the work of druggists and midwives.

There are in present Hungary 318 medical officers and 932 communal (township) and district doctors, who represent the hygienic and medical care of the community. Every commune having a population of 600 must maintain a midwife, or a larger number in proportion to population.

Centrally, public health and medical matters are controlled by the Ministry of Public Welfare and Labour, Dr. Joseph Vass being the Minister, and Dr. Scholtz, already mentioned, the Executive State Secretary. The Ministry is divided into

[1] About 81 per cent. of death certificates are now given by qualified medical practitioners.

a number of departments, of which the following may be mentioned:

1. Department of General and Social Hygiene.
2. Department for Provision for the Sick Hospitals, Dispensaries, Nursing, etc.
3. Workers' Insurance Department.
4. Department for Child Protection and Care of War-Orphans.
5. Public Charity Department.
6. Housing Department.
7. Department of the Hygienic Institutes.

It will be convenient to describe first the two hygienic institutes in Budapest.

THE INSTITUTE AND MUSEUM OF SOCIAL HYGIENE

The Institute and Museum of Social Hygiene, of which Dr. Georg Gortvay is the Sectional Councillor, has existed since 1901 as a sociological museum, including the famous collection of models, etc., illustrating the popular errors of quackery, which were so greatly admired at the International Hygienic Congress at Dresden. The museum contains now an admirable collection of illustrations of the various phases of hygiene, including its industrial application. Since 1927 it has been taken over by the Government, and is now, like the Hygienic Institute, under the Minister of Public Welfare and Labour. At this institute advice on hygienic matters is given, lectures and demonstrations to workers and to scholars are organised, data on hygienic propaganda are collected, and in various other ways the institute is an important centre of enlightenment and of research into the social aspects of health and disease. Its utility in the latter respect could, I think, be greatly extended—to the common advantage of the two institutes and of the entire country—were this institute and the Hygienic Institute to become so closely related as to have a single impetus and outlook. The Institute of Social Hygiene is not yet fully equipped in personnel, etc., to enable it to undertake all the important work in social hygiene which is needed.

STATE HYGIENIC INSTITUTE

The *State Hygienic Institute*, like the State Institute of Social Hygiene, is admirably housed, though unfortunately the two are not in the same part of Budapest. In the absence of Dr. B. Johan, the Director of the Hygienic Institute, I saw every department of the institute in the company of Dr. J. Tomesik and Dr. Mitchell. The institute has a building of which it may be proud; and there is no doubt that the future progress of public health in Hungary will be largely wrapped up in the welfare and uninterrupted progress of scientific work in the two institutes—of Hygiene and Social Hygiene—which Hungary already possesses. The general scope of the work of the Hygienic Institute may be gathered from the scheme on facing page. There is a large site adjoining the institute on which it is proposed to build a nurses' home and training-school as part of the institute. An institute for research on cancer is also to be built on the same site. As will be seen from the scheme, epidemiology is not yet a separate course of study; and both in this department—now to be developed—in the nursing section, and also in statistics, it is evident that combined activity of the two institutes would be advantageous.

But already much epidemiological and administrative work is being done by the Hygienic Institute for the State. The institute has replaced a former Government Bacteriological Laboratory, and not only are very many bacteriological and serological diagnoses made in it, but also gratuitous services have been organised for Hungary as a whole in public health laboratories. There are now seven of these. By recent Government regulations it has been enacted that the use of these laboratories shall be compulsory! Thus every physician notifying a case of diphtheria or typhoid fever, or possibly typhus or plague, will be under an obligation to send an appropriate pathological specimen from the case reported.

The institute has a section for testing and standardising sera and pharmaceutical preparation; and anyone proposing to advertise a patent drug must first obtain a certificate

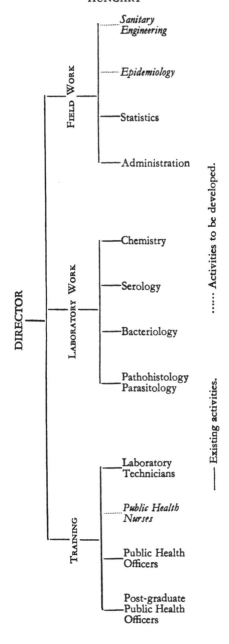

from the Ministry of Public Welfare that the composition and claims of the preparation are in accordance with the claims made for it. Many advertised drugs have been withdrawn as the result of this regulation.

Every druggist throughout Hungary is obliged to keep sera for the treatment of disease, according to a specified list, ready for any physician in emergencies. The Hygienic Institute does not manufacture these preparations, but undertakes their standardisation. The sera, etc., are supplied free for the use of the poor; others pay in accordance with regulated prices.

The Hygienic Institute has an important teaching department, which will include in the future the training of nurses. For some years health officers in Hungary have been required to undergo a three months' course of special instruction. This has been taken over by the institute and lengthened to nine months, during which students obtain a good training in the scientific side of hygiene. The number of students is limited to twenty-four; all of these go into the governmental or local health services.

It should be added that the Central Government hands over a considerable proportion of the work of the public health service, not only in laboratory work, but also often in the investigation of epidemics, and in advising on various public health problems, to the Hygienic Institute. *De facto* if not *de jure* the Hygienic Institute, like the Institute of Social Hygiene, is a technical branch of the Ministry of Social Welfare.

The chief object of my investigation being to ascertain the relation of private members of the medical profession to the various local and central public health and medical activities, it will be convenient to discuss this subject under the various headings of—

1. Number of Doctors in the Community.
2. Provision for the Treatment of the Sick Poor.
3. Midwifery Provision.
4. The National Medical Insurance System.
5. Provision for Care of Mothers and Infants.

6. Provision for Older Children.
7. Provision for Tuberculosis.
8. Provision for Venereal Diseases.

These are the chief subjects in which this relation presents problems of general interest.

DISTRIBUTION OF PHYSICIANS, ETC.

In 1926 there were 5,850 physicians in Hungary, or 0·7 per 1,000 of population. In 1929 there were 7,165, or 0·8 per 1,000 of population. In Budapest the proportion of physicians in these two years was 2·8 and 3·2 per 1,000. The number of druggists in 1924 was 1,163; in 1926, 1,328. In 1921 there were 5,834 midwives; in 1926, 6,048.

There is an excessive supply of doctors in Hungary, but these are very unequally distributed. Owing to the obligation common to Hungary, Italy, France, and Jugo-Slavia, to provide a doctor for each commune, there is nowhere an absolute absence of medical aid. There is, however, the same tendency as is seen, for instance, in New York State, for the doctors to aggregate chiefly in urban centres, and especially in the larger towns. The majority of the doctors are in towns, the minority in rural districts, although the rural population is some six million, the urban population some two million people. The earnings of doctors are extremely meagre, about which more will be said in later paragraphs. This position is mitigated slightly by the system under which "employed doctors", i.e. those in the service of the State, either in the public health or insurance work, receive a pension. A scheme for this purpose has recently come into operation, also for private doctors, towards which the State contributes.

MIDWIFERY PROVISION

For much of the information given below I am indebted to Captain Norvath, the Secretary of the Institute and Museum of Social Hygiene. For many years the practice of midwives has been regulated. Thus a law passed in 1876, while allowing existing midwives to continue practice, required all future midwives to secure a certificate of competency, or failing this, to satisfy the medical officer of the district in which they proposed to practise that they were qualified for the work. The certificate was made compulsory for all women living not more than 75 km. (about 57 miles) distant from a training-school for mid-wives. It was also provided that any midwife licensed as above by a medical officer must discontinue practice—unless within two years she obtained a certificate of competency—if a certified midwife settled in the district. Municipalities were forbidden by Article 51 of the above law to employ any other than certified midwives.

The law required that every community with 1,500 inhabitants must employ a midwife, other smaller communes joining to employ one. Salaries are fixed according to a scale. The midwife, outside her salary, for which she attends the poor gratuitously, must accept the fees fixed by the council of the commune in which she lives. The county medical officer is responsible for the control of the midwives in the communes within the county.

Later laws were passed in 1878 and 1879, as to professional secrecy, and providing for the punishment of doctors or midwives who refused to give the help called for. The notification of infectious diseases was required, and midwives were precluded from certain occupations, as, for instance, anything concerned with putrid matters or the laying out of the dead.

By an Order of 1896 midwives were required to notify each birth within twenty-four hours to the local registrar, oral intimations (possibly to a magistrate, when the distance to the registrar was great) being substituted if the midwife was illiterate. In 1902 laws were codified and extended. Any disciplinary action exercised by the health officer or the district doctor must be entered on each occasion in a booklet kept for this purpose by each midwife. Thus medical control includes the method of distribution and use of pastilles of mercuric chloride. The health officer is required and the district doctor is entitled to exercise this control.

A midwife desiring to settle in a district is required to submit her certificates to the health officer, and to report her settlement to the local magistrate. We need not detail the exact restrictions given to her, which include the sending for medical aid in the complications of parturition and in sickness. She is not allowed to undertake any sick nursing, especially if there are wounds. The doctor to be sent for can be chosen by the patient, if she can pay.

By the law of 1908 it was made compulsory for every commune with a population of 800 to employ a midwife qualified by training in a school of midwives. A few partially trained midwives remain, but these are rapidly being replaced by midwives who have had a two years' training. This training is paid for by the State, but the midwife undertakes to remain for five years practising in the commune to which she is allotted. Midwifery in the main is an official practice, the income derivable from paying patients being small. It is only in a small proportion of total confinements that medical aid is invoked.

For larger communities one official midwife must be provided for every 5,000 inhabitants. If a commune makes default in this respect, the prefect can appoint a midwife, debiting her salary to local funds. In towns midwives are appointed by the municipal council or council of aldermen, in small areas by the local magistrate.

The midwives are required to attend post-graduate courses of instruction; the expense of this, like that of the training of midwives, is borne by the State.

The use of a silver solution is required as a routine measure for the prevention of ophthalmia neonatorum.

The salaries of midwives are 400 to 600 pengös per annum. They can charge 8 to 16 pengös per patient (including also puerperal care) to those patients who are not poor.

In 1922 the Government sent out a circular letter urging local authorities to increase the pitifully small salaries at present paid to midwives. This is an incidental illustration of the low payment given for all professional work, and naturally leads to some remarks on—

The Economic Condition of Hungary

which has made this almost inevitable. The same cause has undoubtedly hastened the maturation of the national scheme of Insurance for Sickness. Provision for medical attendance in sickness (irrespective of sickness allowances) is a first need of civilised mankind. The mass of the people in Hungary could not afford it. Hence the national system of insurance of medical attendance for all employed persons, which is rendered practicable even in present circumstances by the willingness of the doctors—advised by their combinations or syndicates—to accept terms of payment which are much too low, and which must inevitably be raised when Hungary's financial position improves.

Nearly 70 per cent. of the population of Hungary are peasants. In each of the ten wards of the capital city of Budapest about 24 per cent. of the population are treated in illness by the district or poor law medical officer. In order to secure this aid approximately one-fourth of the population are registered in the official poverty record; and when required must show their "poor paper" to the doctor, when visiting his consulting-room or when applying for a doctor at home.

In its present restricted area Hungary has little indigenous coal and no iron. Work is cheap and workers over-abundant, but occupations are limited, and there is no staple industry except agriculture, in which about 70 per cent. of the population are engaged. Not only is payment of industrial labour very low, but the middle and professional classes now are not very far above this level. Some of the figures as to the remuneration of the staff in Universities in the four national Universities given me are almost incredible. There are three ranks at the University from which my figures were obtained. The University Professor gets a maximum salary of 500–600 pengös a month, the Assistant Professor 240 pengös, an Associate 120 pengös a month, from which is deducted the cost of room and board. (100 pengös = £3 15s., or nearly 19 dollars.) On these salaries they are expected to live and maintain the standard of their position.

A sidelight is thrown on the subject by a statement by Assistant Professor B. Kovrig, writing in *Tàrsadalombiztosîtàsi Közlöny* (April 1929). He discusses the general complaint made as to the cost of the insurance contributions, and gives the relation of these payments to the average wage. This average wage is given as 1,102.4 pengös annually (a little over £41 a year). He concludes that, with the exception of Italy, all the States which may be regarded as industrially competitive with Hungary pay higher charges for social insurance (including sickness, accident, invalidity, old age) than is paid in Hungary.

CONTRIBUTION STATED AS A PERCENTAGE OF WORKMEN'S
WAGE IN DIFFERENT COUNTRIES (KOVRIG)

Hungary	10·58
Germany	14·91
Austria	17·60
England	5·80[1]
Czecho-Slovakia	10·72
Italy	8·12

It is no exaggeration to state that the majority of clerks, shop-assistants, typists, and even shopkeepers, as well as a very high proportion of professional workers, are not now able to pay for satisfactory medical attendance, unless a system of insurance can be provided for them. That they will all be included in such a system ere long appears to be inevitable. The inclusion of the agriculturists who are not employed by others is imminent.

The remuneration of doctors is extremely inadequate. It does not suffice to blame the system of National Sickness Insurance for this. Such an attribution of responsibility argues an imperfect and partially erroneous analysis of

[1] 42 per cent. of the cost of social insurance in England is paid by the State. The above comparisons do not include unemployment insurance. I cannot vouch for their exact comparability.

national circumstances in Hungary. To blame insurance for the present financial position of Hungarian doctors is less accurate than it would be to state that in the absence of insurance, either the vast majority of the insured would go untreated, or the doctors would treat them without payment. But would not the poor in such a case be treated by the poor-law doctor? Some of them might, but the salaries received by these doctors are so inadequate, and the standard of work is so low, that—as an alternative to insurance—it cannot be regarded with complacency. The district doctors for treatment of the poor are paid 240 pengös a month (about £9, or $45).

INSURANCE FOR SICKNESS

Austria, in 1888, followed the example given by Germany, in 1883–88, in social insurance. In 1891 a similar system was applied to Hungary for accidents. In 1901 Hungary adopted the principle of compulsory insurance, and constituted a single national organ for carrying this out. In this scheme the burden of sickness insurance was thrown equally on employers and employees, arrangements being made for their equal representation in the administration of the scheme. The burden of accident insurance was thrown solely on the employers. The genesis of new private insurance organisations was prevented; and the unified scheme made for equal control and benefit throughout the country. From the beginning the Hungarian scheme provided medical treatment for the family of the insured, without any separate payment for this benefit.

After the Great War an impetus was given to social insurance in Hungary, as a bulwark against Bolshevism, and the Hungarian insurance scheme developed much more rapidly than the public health organisation, with which it should go hand-in-hand.

By the Act of 1927 all persons of either sex or any nationality who "render services for wages" must be insured against sickness. This includes not merely industrial occupations, but also clerks, shop-assistants, police, and many others employed for wages. Workers in industrial and transport enterprises are insured, whatever their wages; officials, overseers, etc., need not be insured if their income exceeds 3,600 pengös a year (£135). Very few are exempted by this limit.

The dues for sickness insurance paid by the workman or employee amount to 6 per cent. of his actual earnings, an equal amount being paid by the employer. The monetary allowance for a year during a member's sickness from the fourth day onward is 60 per cent. of his average daily wage. In the event of death a burial aid of thirty times the deceased's daily wage is given. Medical treatment is given for a year after falling ill, including the items detailed below.

An insured female when pregnant receives an allowance during six weeks before and six weeks after her confinement, equal to what would be the aggregate of her total daily wages during this period. She receives the attendance of a midwife, and of a doctor also, if necessary. For twelve weeks after the confinement she is given three-fifths of a pengö, or about 5d. a day, if she suckles her infant; double this amount for twins. Milk may also be granted as a supplementary aid during pregnancy or afterwards, and sometimes an outfit of baby-linen. She may have further aid if, on the certificate of a doctor, she is required to stay at home to nurse her sick child.

Members of the insured person's family also receive free medical treatment; and in the event of childbirth monetary aid almost equal to that given to the insured female.

The medical benefit for insured and their relatives alike includes medical treatment, drugs, and appliances for a year, in the case of persons who have been insured during two years, and hospital treatment during a period of four weeks. The family, unlike the insured person, are not entitled to special baths or sanatorium treatment, or to funeral aid. Some nursing aid is given.

When ill the insured person, or any member of his family, visits the doctor allotted to the district in which the patient lives, or, if too ill, sends for the doctor to visit him at

home. The name of the doctor to whom he is allotted can be
ascertained by the patient at any druggist's shop.

Conditions of Engagement and Work of Doctors.—Most of the
particulars on this question I obtained in conference with
Dr. Pfeiffer, the Assistant Medical Director of the entire
Insurance Institute. There is no free choice of doctor by
the patient. In every district in Hungary a doctor is allotted
to and lives in the area in which he is responsible for the
medical care of the local insured persons. As in Hungary,
25 per cent. of the population, and in Budapest 80 per cent.
of the population, are insured (altogether over two millions);
and as the rest of the population in the main are poor, it
may be said that the family physician has almost disappeared.
He may reappear if economic conditions greatly improve.
The greater part of the medical treatment of the industrial
and urban population, omitting the imperfect arrangements
for the destitute, is in the charge of insurance doctors.

The entire medical arrangements are centralised and
controlled from the *Central Insurance Institute* in Budapest.
This magnificent edifice, with its vast administrative staff
and its polyclinics for many diseases always open, impresses
one deeply as a masterly organisation, though one could
not avoid the impression that administration was over-
centralised, and that perhaps the head of the organism was
larger than was justified by the size of the body and the
number of its limbs.

The query also arose as to whether, notwithstanding the
admirable arrangements made, the provision was adequate
for unhurried diagnosis and treatment; and whether all
that could be done was being done to avoid prolonged
and uneconomical waiting of patients.

The Central Institute has associated with it thirty-five
branch institutes in various parts of the country, which
reproduce on a smaller scale the general arrangements of
the Central Institute. Each comprises a—

Chief physician,
Deputy chief physician,
Controlling physicians,

Revising physicians,
Specialists for accidents,
Leading specialists for the dispensaries (ambulatories),
Specialists for the dispensaries (ambulatories),
Assistant specialists for the dispensaries (ambulatories),
Clinical physicians for the districts,
Obstetricians for the districts,
Assistant physicians for the districts.

In addition, there are central and district medical advisory and consulting boards, consisting of persons elected from the above officers by the officers themselves.

At Budapest there are 160 doctors in its several institutes in twenty ambulatories or dispensaries. Each of these ambulatories has specialists who deal with—

Special conditions relating to mothers and their infants,
Internal medicine,
Psychopathy,
Gynæcology and obstetrics,
Surgery,
Ophthalmology,
Ear, nose, and throat cases,
X-ray diagnosis,
Laboratory work,
Zenden exercises.

There is at the Central Institute a magnificent outfit for the dental treatment of the insured and their families. Here not only extractions and stoppings are made gratuitously, but also dentures are provided on the same terms when medically recommended. This department was shown me by Dr. Csillery, former Minister of Health, now the head of the Government Department for dental treatment. Under his charge the work is rapidly growing. Already the numbers treated are phenomenally large, and the value of dental treatment clearly is becoming widely recognised.

Ambulatories.—The records of the ambulatoria show that, on an average, a doctor consults with 13·5 patients a day. Each physician attends 1 to 1½ hours; at the dental clinics, 3 hours.

Statistics for the year 1922 showed that during the year 147,634 insured patients came under a doctor's care. For men this works out at 24·6 and for women 18·6 per cent. of the respective insured persons.

Distribution and Payment of Doctors.—As already stated, there is no free choice of doctor. For domiciliary treatment and consultations at the doctor's office it is arranged that the doctor shall not have more than 1,000 members in his area. In general his salary amounts to about 6 pengös a year for each insured person. The salary is not computed on a *per capita* basis, but an index number is ascertained, based on area and the number of persons to be served.

In all areas in which there are treatment centres or ambulatories, part-time doctors are appointed who may work for 1, 2, or 3 hours daily. The salary paid for this is 100 pengös for each daily hour of work during a month (or £45 per annum). If the doctor attends in the afternoon, when he might otherwise see private patients, he is paid 50 per cent. more for each hour's work. Outside Budapest similar work is paid for at the monthly rate of 60 to 80 pengös per hour of daily work.

Supervisory Doctors.—The home work of each district doctor is overlooked by a *supervisory doctor.* This system of supervision was inaugurated two years ago. The supervisor visits weekly every patient who is under the care of a district doctor. In doing so, he not only checks excessive claims for sickness benefit, but also acts as a consultant and as a medium through which specialist or hospital help is obtained to a larger extent than formerly. The supervisory doctors are engaged on a whole-time basis. In Budapest there are some 700 ordinary insurance doctors and 45 supervisory doctors.

Engagement of Doctors.—This is a matter of great difficulty. Although the remuneration offered is on a scale admittedly too low, there is much competition for vacant positions. The difficulty for the Insurance Institute is overcome by the appointment of a self-governing Medical Advisory Board, who, except its president, are elected by the doctors already employed by the institute. This board is entrusted with two delicate tasks: (*a*) the appointment of new medical officers; (*b*) the decision as to whether the number of medical officers shall be increased in proportion to a given number of insured persons.

The operations of this board are subject to the conditions of a basic contract entered between the Central Insurance Institute and the General Association of Physicians of Hungary, as representing the organised medical profession of the country. This contract is based on the reservation of a fixed proportion of the total income obtained from insurance premiums for the payment of doctors. This has been fixed at 11·5 per cent., including the salaries of the doctors working in the central clinics. The total amount available thus fixed for medical work compares with 17 per cent. of the total expenditure which is required for central and local administration. The question arises as to whether the cost of centralised administration might not be reduced. On this point I cannot give more than a hesitant opinion. But a long experience of official life has shown me the need for drastic and meticulous guarding against unnecessary multiplication of administrative posts, as well as the avoidance of salaries which range too high in proportion to those of the doctors who do the vital work of the institute.

In existing circumstances the problem for the Medical Advisory Board is one of distribution of the allotted money. There is a constant pressure to appoint new doctors, while those already engaged in the work do not favour this, as every addition means a lowered income for those already engaged in the work. Generally, doctors are appointed in open competition by the Medical Advisory Board. The Central Advisory Board consists of twenty-four members, and the corresponding board in each county has numbers in proportion to the number of insured. Doctors already employed cannot be dismissed, except by a judicial committee on which doctors are represented.

It is evident from the above that the Medical Advisory

Board is the "buffer" between the Insurance Institute and the medical profession. To improve the relations between doctors and the insurance administration the large sum recently granted for pensions for doctors may be regarded as a useful contribution.

It should be added that, although most of the insurance doctors are engaged on a part-time basis, their earnings outside their official work are almost negligible. In an interesting interview with Dr. Kovrig, the official head of the Insurance Department of the Government, I gathered many hints as to the general policy of the insurance organisation. Although some points overlap with what has already been stated, a summary of my impression from the interview is permissible at this point.

It is claimed that a centralised system, without conflicting or competitive societies, gives much economy in administration and opens the way for great future developments in preventive medicine. The unification of the machinery for sickness, for accidents, for old age and survivors, and for invalidity is an important feature of the Hungarian system; and the medical service for all these schemes is similarly unified. The method of dealing collectively, in respect of 2,200 "employed doctors," with the Association of Hungarian Physicians is noteworthy. It is held that the main interest is that of the insured; and it is agreed that this may mean some hardship for the medical profession. The dilemma of the representatives of the medical profession is realised. The larger the number of doctors employed beyond what is needed for efficient service, the less in the national circumstances must be the remuneration of the individual doctor; for in these circumstances it is not possible to increase the weekly payments of workers or masters, even if these were not fixed by Parliament. Actuarial considerations forbid the allotment of a larger proportion of the total insurance expenditure to medical expenses.

In a private interview another physician voiced another view of medical insurance. In his opinion it is the honest man who suffers under this system. Conscientious care is not rewarded on its merits. Many insured patients seek supplementary advice from private doctors, who treat the patient and not only his disease. I was not impressed greatly by this viewpoint. In both private and insurance medical work there are many opportunities for careless and indifferent work and for medical quackery. The conditions of employment—salaried, or paid per attendance—need not essentially or necessarily modify medical attendance, and conscientious and intelligent work may not be more general under one than under the other system.

Nor was I impressed with the criticism expressed in another quarter, that the medical insurance system represented "mediocrity enthroned". Evidently the expert consultative and clinical services at the ambulatories, the facilities for pathological diagnosis, the access to hospital treatment, etc., mean a great advance on pre-existing conditions and an advance which could not otherwise have been attained, except by a national system of gratuitous State medicine.

It appears clear that in the present circumstances of Hungary its medical men would not benefit—but would lose—by abolition of sickness insurance. Some improvement in medical conditions may be looked for with economic recovery. If agriculturists and others are included in the scheme, some improvement will result from diminution of overhead administrative expenses. There would be a more hopeful prospect if greater energy were devoted to the promotion of social hygiene and improved public health administration.

Hungary is a poor country, and voluntary effort counts for little in social and hygienic improvement. There is great need for the development of social sentiment.

Attitude of the Medical Profession.—The medical profession is represented by the National Association of Physicians. With its president, Dr. Csillery, I had the advantage of conferring. Like other physicians, he has appreciated the inevitableness of the great medical changes which have occurred, and, as already mentioned, is now the responsible head for the section of insurance work dealing with the dental treatment of the insured and their families. The growth of this dental work has been phenomenal. Dental service is rendered gratuitously and—as I have found in other countries, and as is experienced in Britain—gratuitous dental service is sanctioned and accepted without any considerable difficulty from the side of either dentists or doctors.

Dr. Csillery expounded the general position of the medical profession, as represented by its National Association. They do not favour medical insurance; they dislike a system which does not permit each patient to select his own doctor. Their objection to insurance is based chiefly on the absence of this free choice. I gathered that they appreciate, nevertheless, that the districted system of medical attendance on the insured and their families is preferable from the standpoint of economy of effort and expense; and they realise that the expert and hospital services made possible under the insurance system would not in Hungary be practicable apart from this, except on a gratuitous basis, paid for by the State. Hence the general attitude of the medical profession appears to be that medical insurance must be accepted; and it appears to be appreciated that in the present national circumstances of Hungary the too meagre remuneration offered by this service is perhaps better than would be received if the insurance service did not exist.

RELATION OF INSURANCE TO PUBLIC HEALTH

It appears to me that to some extent medical insurance has "shot ahead" at the expense of preventive medicine and its application in public health measures. This was almost inevitable, in view of the immediate need to secure adequate skilled medical aid for all wage-earners. But, nevertheless, the incompleteness of public health work and the imperfections of the liaison between public health authorities and the insurance organisation are regrettable. The defect is realised, and the remedy will be applied. The possibilities of early fusion of the two activities, or at least of closer collaboration, already exist, for the areas of the local insurance organisations have been made mostly coterminous with county administrative areas. In some localities there is unfriendliness between the two public agencies; in others the position is one of passive inactivity; in a few there is close co-operation. The Insurance Institute evidently has vast prophylactic ambitions; but they can only be satis-factorily and permanently realised if every local sanitary authority takes the leading part in the practical measures of prophylaxis which are needed.

MATERNITY AND CHILD WELFARE WORK

The national arrangement for providing official mid-wives in every commune has already been indicated. In other respects most of the work hitherto directed to pro-moting the welfare of the mother and infant has been in the hands of a voluntary but semi-official society. More recently the Insurance Institute is occupying some of this ground.

The system of birth registration is similar to that in England, and the following birth-rates and rates of infant mortality may be regarded as fairly reliable.

The birth-rate for the whole of present Hungary in 1921–25 was 29·4, in 1929 it was 24·1, per 1,000 of popula-tion. In the past, Hungary has had one of the highest birth-rates in Europe. Now the "one-child system" is becoming increasingly prevalent. The rate of infant mor-tality in 1929 was 182 per 1,000 live-births. It had been 198 in 1922, and so far there is only small evidence of decline in this delicate index of child-health for the whole country. For Budapest the record is more satisfactory, as shown in the diagram on page 196, which gives also the death-rate for infants under a month old.

The *Stephanie Federation* was established in 1916 for organising measures for the protection of mothers and infants, and was recognised by the then Royal Hungarian Government as the organ for carrying out this part of the duty of the State. It has among its points of policy one which will appeal to child-lovers, viz. that no mother should sink into a worse economic condition as the result of giving birth to a new citizen. It has a large central organisation with some 190 branch establishments or

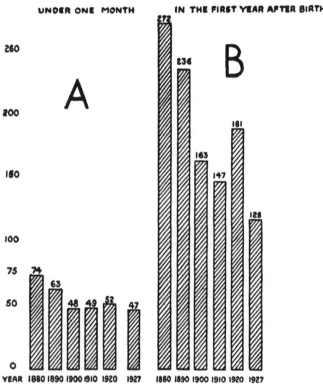

dispensaries throughout the country, at which mothers and infants receive medical guidance. There are ten of these in Budapest. No treatment is carried out at the dispensaries, except rarely. Patients requiring treatment are referred to a doctor or hospital. The doctors in charge of each dispensary are local practising physicians, except those for antenatal clinics, which are usually served by specialists. They receive the sum of 50–70 pengös for a month's attendance at the clinic, sometimes daily! (a pengö = 9d.). The State contributed last year 1,200,000 pengös towards this work: and the work is not usually objected to by private doctors, as the mothers attending the clinics are poor, and treatment is not given. Each dispensary receives notification of local births either daily or weekly. This registration is not required for eight days after birth, and two or three days more elapse before the visiting nurse receives the notice. The amount of home visiting varies greatly in different areas. The nurses of the federation do not pay home visits for other branches of health work than child welfare. Altogether in 1928 the nurses made 81,802 visits, and it is estimated that mothers and infants representing 20 per cent. of the total births in Hungary received help from the federation.

The Central Institute in Budapest serves for the administration of the work of the federation throughout Hungary. It has also a school and home for nurses, with fifty-five residential students and forty non-resident. Free teaching and training, with board, is given to these nurses at the expense of the federation, on the condition that they work during two years in its service on a paid salary.

The training includes maternity nursing, and the Central Institute has lying-in wards with twenty-one beds. These are intended for the poor, who are received for six weeks gratuitously. There is also a prenatal clinic, at which there is a large attendance. The nurses receive their practical training in the hospital, and also in other divisions of the institute in which an infant consultation is held daily, and there are beds and cots for infants needing special in-patient treatment. Children attend the consultation up to the age of 3 years. During the first year they attend fortnightly with their mothers, and only a small proportion fail to do this. Usually half a litre of milk is given daily, for the mother or for her infant. It is stated that in Budapest about 60 per cent. of all babies born attend the Stephanie Federation's dispensaries, of which there are twenty-one in the city.

The Central Insurance Institute profits by the work of the Stephanie Federation, as do also the Public Health Authorities. Between the three some measure of joint working has been secured, and sometimes the Insurance Institute contributes to the funds of the federation as a return for its work, especially in the supply of nurses. It is evident, however, that in regard to this, as to other branches of work in social hygiene, there is need for a revision of methods as well as for extension of work if the greatest good is to be secured for the public from the at present unsatisfactorily related work of the Stephanie Federation, Public Health Authorities, and the Insurance Institutes. These relationships are improving, but much more needs to be done.

CARE OF OLDER CHILDREN

These, like infants, if in an insured family, are entitled to medical care. But the above independent organisation continues and is utilised largely for the infants in insured families; and for the pre-school child, and still more for the scholar, there is also some—true it is a very imperfect —medical provision outside the insurance scheme.

Some of the following particulars are taken from a written statement by Dr. A. Bexhaft, school physician at Budapest. The idea of instituting school physicians for every elementary school initiated with the late Dr. F. Fodor, Professor of Hygiene in the University of Budapest, who, as financial resources were inadequate, proposed to begin with the high schools, thus promoting the interest of the pupils in health matters. This was organised in 1885. Now most high schools in the metropolis have a school physician, and at last the same can be said for the elementary schools. If a parent objects to his child being examined by the school doctor, he is required to obtain such an examination from a private doctor, who informs the school director of his findings.

The school doctor is required to give popular hygienic addresses at intervals. He must not treat the pupils found to need treatment. An exception is made for dental treatment, which is given gratuitously with the consent of the parent. School nurses attend the doctors in their inspections of pupils, and visit the homes of those needing treatment.

TUBERCULOSIS WORK

Tuberculosis causes a very heavy mortality in Hungary. In 1910, with a population of 18¼ millions, the tuberculosis death-rate was 3·4; in 1925 its population of 8 millions experienced a death-rate of 2·6 per 1,000. In Budapest, in 1910, the corresponding death-rate was 3·6, and in 1925 it was 3·1.

There is no unified national anti-tuberculosis campaign for the whole of Hungary. No voluntary associations devote themselves especially to this work. Voluntary associations —apart from the Stephanie Federation, which is semi-official—do not flourish. It may almost be said that only State efforts succeed, the chief among these being the Insurance Institutes. At these there are special clinics for tuberculosis and venereal diseases; sputa are examined freely for all coming within the scheme, and the insurance scheme supports sanatoria, etc. Altogether about fifty clinics have been recently started in connection with the Insurance Institutes for consumptives; but little "field work" is done from these, and the regrettable deficiency of practical co-operation between public health and insurance authorities, noted in other paragraphs, is very serious in regard to this disease.

The Stephanie Federation also includes anti-tuberculosis work in its child welfare activities. The municipality of Budapest has erected several large institutes or hospitals for the treatment of tuberculous patients, and such patients are also treated at the University clinics. There are also two large sanatoria at Budakeszi and Gyula, which receive subventions from the State. The total efforts made are unequal to the need. In particular there is pressing need for the hospital treatment of advanced and bedridden consumptives: and a much more active campaign, persistent and continuous, is needed to educate the people into more hygienic habits, especially as regards coughing and expectoration. This, in particular, is an instance in which combined and unremitting effort by the Insurance Institutes and by the Public Health Authorities would, ere long, bear fruit in reduced expenses for the maintenance of the destitute and for sickness benefits to the insured.

Venereal Diseases

The best work in regard to these diseases is being done at the four University clinics of Hungary and in one or two additional centres. Free treatment is given to patients in clinics at the four Universities of Budapest, Debreczen, Pécs, and Szeged; and this treatment, like the rest of the University work, is supported by the Government. At the polyclinics of the Insurance Institutes there are clinics for venereal disease for insured persons and their families.

I paid a short visit to Ujpest, a town bordering on Budapest, where there is active anti-venereal work. On the same premises there is also an anti-tuberculosis clinic: and there are other social activities, including lectures, demonstrations, etc., on social and economic subjects.

CHAPTER VI

POLAND[1]

PRELIMINARY SUMMARY

All medico-social work is necessarily of recent origin. Some sickness insurance schemes were inherited from the countries out of which the new Poland was constituted. These systems are now unified in a single organisation, which avoids local or other overlappings. All employed persons must be insured. Domiciliary medical aid is given under several methods.

The outstanding feature of Polish medical insurance, as also of those of Hungary and Czecho-Slovakia, is the enormous development of ambulatories or polyclinics, which are very prone to be excessively used.

The views of the medical profession on this and other medico-social problems are given by Drs. Falkowski and Zaluska for the Polish Medical Union.

The active work of health centres is noteworthy. So also is the position of anti-alcoholic work at clinics and otherwise.

No more enlightening view of social conditions in Poland could be rapidly obtained than by a drive in an automobile through the country from Breslau to Warsaw, which I experienced in the latter part of May 1929. One could not fail to be impressed by the vast extent of Polish territory, its apparently interminable plains, in the cultivation of which women play a prominent part, by the squalor of its villages and hamlets, by the defects of its roads, becoming steadily worse as one passed from the former German to the former Russian Poland, and by the general evidence of a low standard of life in the countryside. Even in the prolonged outskirts of Lodz and of Warsaw one was impressed by the evidence of poverty and of deplorable housing; and only when the more central parts of Warsaw were reached did one begin fully to realise that side by side with these

[1] Date of investigation, May 1929.

evidences of impoverishment there were noble buildings, wide streets, and a large population possessed of high culture as well as of most fervid patriotism.

As independent Poland only dates from after the Great War, its public health and medical arrangements in their present form are in their infancy; and the present attainment, therefore, is surprising.

In 1921, Poland as now constituted had a population of 27½ millions, of whom 69·2 per cent. were Polish and 31·8 per cent. belonged to other nationalities. This 31·8 per cent. was made up as follows: Of the total population, 14·3 per cent. were Ruthenes, 7·8 per cent. Jews, 3·9 per cent. White Ruthenes, 3·8 per cent. Germans, with smaller proportions of Lithuanians, Russians, and Czechs.

Reference to a map will show the position of Poland in Central Europe. Westward is Germany; on the north are the free town of Dantzig, and Eastern Prussia, Lithuania and Lettonia; on the east is Soviet Russia; and on the south Roumania and Czecho-Slovakia.

Poland is a republic, its President being elected for a period of seven years. Its legislative body consists of two chambers, a Lower Chamber (Sejm) consisting of 444 deputies, and a Senate of 111 senators. There is universal suffrage, on a proportional basis, to ensure representation of minorities. The Government has a Council of fourteen ministers.

(Democratic government has been partially suspended since the above paragraph was written.)

The country is divided into 16 provinces (voievodies). Of these, 4 represent Austrian territory, 3 Prussian, and 9 Russian territory of the past. Each voievodie is divided into districts. The number of districts in a voievodie and their population varies greatly.

It is not proposed to describe in full the local governmental methods of Poland. They are too recent to furnish useful lessons. The following particulars refer to special work I had the opportunity of observing in Warsaw and in Posen.

SCHOOL OF HYGIENE

It will simplify my task if I describe first the organisation of the School of Hygiene in Warsaw, as much of the hope of future progress in health depends on this institution. A fuller description of the work of the school by Dr. W. Chodzko is contained in the monthly bulletin of the Office International d'Hygiène publique (1928, fasc. No. 1).

To Dr. Chodzko, the head of the school, and to members of its staff, especially to Dr. Nowakowski (Dr. Chodzko's deputy), to Dr. Kacprzaka, and his associate, Mme S. Adamowicz, as well as to Dr. Hirschfeld, the director of the institute, I am greatly indebted for the time they devoted to me and for most of the information which follows.

The School of Hygiene is a division of the Institute of Hygiene, and is indebted to the Rockefeller Foundation for its initiation and rapid progress.

The Institute of Hygiene began its work during the great epidemics of 1919, Dr. Rajchman, now of the League of Nations, being its director. Its present fine buildings comprise departments of research and of teaching, organised as shown in the following scheme :—

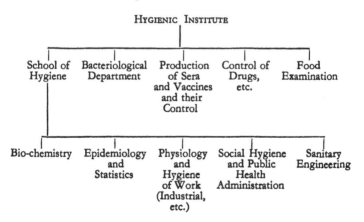

HYGIENIC INSTITUTE

School of Hygiene	Bacteriological Department	Production of Sera and Vaccines and their Control	Control of Drugs, etc.	Food Examination

Bio-chemistry	Epidemiology and Statistics	Physiology and Hygiene of Work (Industrial, etc.)	Social Hygiene and Public Health Administration	Sanitary Engineering

Each of these divisions of the work of the school forms part of the organisation of the institute, and the professor and his auxiliary staff in each division are engaged not only in teaching, but in research work bearing on their special branch of hygiene. Many teachers are also introduced from without, who give special courses of lectures.

The school is used in training officers for the public health service. Any doctor engaged in the governmental part of this service is required to spend a year of probation in the school, in which is included six months' theoretical training in the school and three months' practical work.

He is paid by the State during this period of training. The six months' course of instruction is divided into hours as follows:—

104 in legal medicine, autopsies, etc., of which 100 are practical exercises.
116 bacteriology, immunology, and medical zoology.
238 epidemiology and vital statistics.
68 physiology and hygiene of nutrition.
66 physiology and hygiene of work.
80 sanitary engineering.
70 social hygiene.
70 public health administration.

The three months' practical training is chiefly in the two last-named branches of work. It includes the diagnosis of infectious diseases, attendance at clinics for tuberculosis, venereal disease, trachoma, infant consultations, and practical work at dispensaries for these conditions.

Demonstrations of public health administration are given at the four special organised public districts.

After his nine months' tuition the probationer is subjected to an examination, and at the end of the year to a State examination conducted by the Ministry of Health, most of the professors at the school being on the Board of Examiners.

Each year about twenty-five men undertake this course. It is compulsory for officers in the State service; usually city officers also undertake it. It should be noted that local government in Poland is largely centralised, the Government appointing the health officers for provinces and districts. City appointments and appointments for sub-districts are made locally.

For existing health officers short intensive courses of instruction of four to six weeks are arranged.

The school also has courses of instruction for local engineers in the hygienic aspect of their work.

During their vacations, a three weeks' course of instruction is given to school teachers in methods of teaching hygiene in schools. Teachers come at their own expense, and already 600 teachers have gone through this course.

Special courses in preventive medicine for practising physicians have been arranged.

Schools for Nurses

The above statement shows great future possibilities for public health in Poland. A similar remark applies to the nursing position in Poland, as illustrated in the new Nursing School in Warsaw, only recently opened, which I inspected in the company of Mlle Bablicka, of the Ministry of the Interior, on May 25th. It owes its initiation to a "foundation" in 1921 under the auspices of the Polish and the American Red Cross Societies, the latter giving valuable pecuniary help.

Its present executive board consists of two representatives of the Ministry of the Interior, two of the Ministry of Labour, one of the Ministry of Education, one of Warsaw University, two councillors of the city of Warsaw, one representative of the Polish Red Cross, and one representative elected by the private subscribers.

The Rockefeller Foundation has defrayed half the cost of the handsome buildings. Its upkeep will be provided to the extent of one-third by nurses' payments, one-third by the city, and one-third by other institutions. The curriculum must be endorsed by the Ministry of the Interior. Each pupil costs 250 zlotys (about 123 shillings) per month, and pays towards this amount from 65 zlotys per month and an entrance fee of 125 zlotys. Pupils who do not pay the full cost of their training are required to work for three to five years afterwards. Their pay in nursing is 250 to 400 zlotys per month.

The school is adapted for 100 students. The curriculum lasts two years. Entrants must have passed the examinations of the sixth school-year and be at least 20 years old.

The course of instruction does not differ greatly from that given elsewhere. One-fourth of the time is devoted to theoretical and three-fourths to practical work.

There are five other nurses' schools, among them one Jewish and one for Roman Catholic nuns; but the supply of nurses is still greatly below the national needs, as is incidentally shown by the difficulty at present experienced in obtaining satisfactory teachers for the nurses. In the past the nursing of the sick in hospitals has been done chiefly by religious sisterhoods; and the supply of fully trained nurses remains extremely inadequate. It will be some years before this ceases to be the case.

This deficiency implies that public health nurses are seldom available. To meet the immediate need, young women are being accepted for courses of training in child welfare and tuberculosis work, which last for six months. Thus need has brought about limited specialist training before the generalised training on which it should be based has been secured. In three schools, also, nursemaids are trained, the course for this purpose varying from a half to one year in duration.

A fully trained nurse can get 300 zlotys per month in public health work under municipalities. Private nurses get 15 zlotys per diem.

The above particulars as to training of doctors and nurses throw light on the present position in Poland, and the better prospects for the future. They emphasise the present difficulties in public health and medical progress.

GOVERNMENT

We may now turn to some items of central and local government in Poland. The central control of health problems is in the two departments of the Government, the Ministry of Labour and Social Welfare and the Ministry of the Interior. Public health work is chiefly under the Ministry of the Interior; but the problems of social medicine are under three subdivisions of the

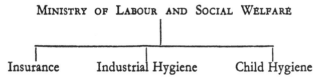

MINISTRY OF LABOUR AND SOCIAL WELFARE

Insurance   Industrial Hygiene   Child Hygiene

In the Industrial Hygiene section about a hundred factory inspectors are employed, for whom courses of instruction are arranged at the School of Hygiene. The chief industry in Poland, outside agriculture, is the manufacture of textiles in Lodz and elsewhere.

Local government is well established under munici-palities in the chief towns. These enjoy some measure of independence of the Government, and they employ their own health officers.

THE SUPPLY OF DOCTORS

The general medical profession is inadequate in numbers for the needs of the population, except possibly in Warsaw. Poland has a much smaller proportion of doctors to population than most Western countries. Their distribution can be seen from the following statement, given me by Professor Kacprzaka, of the School of Hygiene of Poland.

DISTRIBUTION OF DOCTORS IN POLAND, 1928

(Number of Population for One Physician)

Central Provinces	2,700
Eastern Provinces	5,100
Western Provinces	3,500
Southern Provinces	2,700
Poland as a whole	3,100

The distribution of physicians is very unequal, not always following the local standards of culture and finance. This subject is closely related to that of sickness insurance, in which connection further comments will be made.

Medical care is given through *physicians for the destitute*, or by private medical practitioners, or in connection with specialised public health work, or (and chiefly) in the administration of sickness insurance.

Warsaw, with its million people, is divided into five social areas, each having a special part-time doctor for the destitute. These doctors are paid according to the number of hours' work they do.

CHILD HYGIENE CLINICS

Child hygiene clinics may be official or private organisations. The former are often organised at Special Health Centres under the Ministry of the Interior. The national voluntary Committee for the Protection of Child Health has organised about 220 child hygiene stations in Poland, which are commonly subsidised by municipal authorities.

HEALTH CENTRES

In many areas this work is conjoined with that of other branches of social hygiene in *Health Centres*, at which are held consultations for infants and their mothers, and for tuberculosis. Often in the same centres dispensaries are also maintained for alcoholism, for trachoma, and for venereal diseases. For the two last-named diseases it has been found indispensable to provide treatment; for other conditions the watchword has been the maximum of prevention, the minimum of treatment. The conception of health centres is derived from American experience, and its development has been greatly helped by financial aid given to the Health Demonstrations organised with the help of the Rockefeller Foundation.

Already some 150 of these health centres of varying degrees of completeness exist in Poland.

The complete working of a health centre can be seen at the Demonstration Health Centre at Mokotow, a special district of Warsaw with a population of about 54,000. It is under the directorate of Dr. Stypulkowski, who is also M.O.H. for this district.

The centre was initiated in 1925. Its services are limited to the population of this district, of whom about one-third avail themselves of its help. The centre is utilised as a training-ground for the students of the School of Hygiene.

Its activities are directed by a committee comprising representatives of the two Government departments concerned, of the municipality of Warsaw, and of the School of Hygiene and the School of Nursing; and, in addition to the now decreasing Rockefeller grant (given wisely by the Foundation on its usual plan of gradual withdrawal), it is supported by subventions from the Government, the municipality, and the Insurance Fund of Warsaw. In Warsaw the municipality, with the co-operation of the Anti-Tuberculosis Society, has established six similar stations (soon to be increased by two more).

The staff of the Mokotow Health Centre comprises a chief physician (Dr. Stypulkowski), an associate physician, two sanitary inspectors, and a number of specialist physicians, including pediatricians (2), tuberculosis physicians (2), ophthalmologist, laryngologist, alienist, röntgenologist, specialist in malaria (one each), two specialists in venereal diseases, and two dentists. There are twelve public health nurses. These are engaged in the registration and other work of the centre during afternoons, and in the forenoon they pay home visits. The district is divided into ten areas, each nurse having care of one district. Altogether, 2,147 families are cared for by them. All the pupils from the nursing-school are required to work for a time in the anti-alcoholic clinic.

Great importance is attached to the anti-alcoholic clinic, because of the devastating amount of heavy alcoholism which prevails. Under this heading 1,161 home visits and 275 institutional visits were made by the public health nurses. The measures adopted are educational, the medical treatment of dipsomaniacs, and general help conducing to counteract the alcoholic habit. The report of this station[1] emphasises the need for public restrictive measures against this great national evil.

The institute, over which I was conducted by Dr. Stypulkowski, is well planned, and is conducted on admirable lines. An additional building is being added at which baths will be provided at a small charge, and facilities for domestic washing are also being arranged.

Patients coming to the centre are sent by the Insurance Fund, by the Public Assistance, some also by hospitals, and some come as the result of home visits by the nurses. Very few are sent by private doctors. These doctors work almost entirely for the Insurance Fund.

The activities of the centre include a day nursery, to which children under fourteen are admitted. They are given two meals a day, which are supplied free. Mothers fetch their children home at night. For these special children some education is provided at the centre.

Prenatal advice is given at the centre, but mothers are sent elsewhere for attendance in childbirth. Eighty per cent. of the mothers attending the centre belong also to the Sickness Insurance Fund, and a large proportion of these are confined in hospital.

Infant mortality is high, about 160 per 1,000 births. Infants are commonly breast-fed until one year old.

The above is a very incomplete statement of the many activities of this health centre. It should be emphasised that persons coming to it are dealt with from the point of view of a health centre rather than of a dispensary. The exceptions to this rule are the treatment of trachoma and venereal disease, and occasional treatment in other instances.

The outstanding features of the centre are that it is the focus of the activities of the M.O.H. of the district served by it; that its activities are limited to this district; and that in this district it co-ordinates all the public medical activities in one institution.

[1] *Première Station Muncipale d'Hygiène a Mokotow Varsovie*, 1929.

ANTI-TUBERCULOSIS WORK

Anti-tuberculosis work in Poland is directed by the Ministry of the Interior (Department of Health). Educational and propaganda work is largely conducted by the National Anti-Tuberculosis Association. The central committee of this association in Warsaw has on it representatives of the Ministries of the Interior and of Social Welfare, of the city municipality, of the University, and of the Red Cross Society. These choose a national director to organise local organisations, which collect funds and collaborate with the local municipality and with the Central Ministry. It is thought that the local educational work thus secured is some compensation for the lack of uniformity and incompleteness which characterises much local work. The death-rate from tuberculosis in Poland is terribly high.

Actual anti-tuberculosis work centres around dispensaries, which number about 200 in Poland. These sometimes form part of a health centre, sometimes are independent. They may be paid for out of taxes or be voluntary in character.

ANTI-VENEREAL WORK

Some of the larger towns have organised venereal clinics. Most of these are situate in health centres. The ambulatories for sickness insurance also do much of the treatment of venereal diseases. It is in this sphere that the chief friction in Poland between private physicians and public clinics has been experienced. Special objection is taken to the gratuitous administration of arseno-benzol preparations at these clinics. Apparently considerations of expense prevent the objection being met in the right way, by allowing private practitioners to have these preparations gratuitously for their private work.

The treatment of venereal diseases at the insurance ambulatories appears to be thoroughly unsatisfactory. There is no special inducement to secure continuity of treatment, and the conditions under which treatment is given at these ambulatories commonly mean the disappearance of patients as soon as urgent symptoms disappear.

ANTI-ALCOHOLIC EFFORTS

Alcoholism in Poland presents interesting features. There is much anti-alcoholic legislation. No sale of spirits is permitted between Saturday noon and Monday morning. This applies to restaurants; and cocktails are prohibited. The number and position of drinking saloons is regulated. They must not be near a church or school. Any commune objecting to the sale of alcoholic drinks can have local option, and in 165 communes this power has been exercised and total prohibition of sale of alcoholic drinks secured. In sixty-four other communes similar proposals are being made the subject of local voting.

There are six anti-alcoholic dispensaries, some of these at health centres. These are stated to be doing much good. Patients come willingly to them. Good physicians are appointed, who have had three months' training at the School of Hygiene and at a psychiatric hospital.

Alongside this action showing national appreciation of the great seriousness of alcoholism in Poland is the fact —explained by national poverty and the urgent need of revenue—that vodka, the Government monopoly in which ceased with the Russian régime, has once more been restored as such. Its manufacture is limited by the State, only a few manufacturers specially licensed being allowed to produce it (from potatoes and rye). Great profits accrue to the Government from this manufacture. By legislation it is quaintly enacted that 1 per cent. of these profits shall be devoted to anti-alcoholic educational work! Inasmuch as proposals for spending this grant must be approved in detail by the Ministry of Finance, I was informed that the amount actually released for educational work is commonly much smaller than the prescribed quota!

NATIONAL INSURANCE AGAINST SICKNESS

The present law as to compulsory sickness insurance in Poland dates from May 1920. Prior to that date Poland inherited partial insurance systems from the three provinces of which it had consisted for more than a century, under Russia, Prussia, and Austria-Hungary respectively. These provinces differed widely in economic conditions, and the differences persist in a marked degree. In the former Russian province there was in operation compensation for workmen's accidents and insurance of railway employees against accident, as also in State undertakings.

In the former Prussian province the general German Code of 1911, covering insurance against sickness, accident, old age, and for survivors of the insured, held good, as also separate insurance of non-manual workers in private employment (Act of 1911) and Miners' Insurance (Act of 1912). In the former Austria-Hungarian province the position resembled that of the German province. After the war, Poland was left with these systems deeply affecting the life of the people, but with a large part of the accumulated funds gone, and almost completely without competent officials. Then came the evils of depreciation of money. Without attempting to detail the steps taken to make good much of the inherited obligation to the insured, the present position may be briefly sketched, superseding old enactments, except for Upper Silesia.

The Act of 1920 provides for territorial sick funds, each as a rule covering an administrative district. Special funds are permitted in larger cities. Only State employees, including railwaymen, are excepted from the territorial arrangement.

The obligation of insurance for sickness applies to every person, male or female, working under a contract of employment, whatever the occupation and *whatever is the rate of remuneration*. Apprentices, home-workers, and temporary workers are included.

Only State officials nominated to their appointments and the managing directors of industrial and commercial undertakings are exempt. Any person whose annual income does not exceed 7,500 zlotys may become insured.

Contributions.—These are fixed to cover benefits provided for in the rules of the fund. At the beginning they were

6½ per cent. of the basic wage. Contributions must be reduced by funds having small sickness experience, and are increased if there is excessive sickness.

Two-fifths of the contribution is paid by the insured and three-fifths by the employer. For apprentices the entire payment is made by the employer, and voluntary members pay the entire contribution.

State Participation.—The State repays to the sickness funds (*a*) one-half of the money benefits granted to lying-in women and nursing mothers; (*b*) the entire cost of medical assistance to the unemployed or their families; and (*c*) one-half of the milk benefit for infants.

Sick Benefits.—These consist of: (*a*) Free medical attendance, medicine, and some apparatus during 26 weeks, or 39 weeks if the fund has existed over three years. The rules of the fund may provide for extending medical attendance to a maximum of 52 weeks. (*b*) A cash benefit of 60 per cent. of the basic wage for 26 or 39 weeks from the third day of sickness onwards. During hospital treatment members receive one-half of the normal allowance if they have to support members of their family, or 10 per cent. in other cases.

Other Benefits.—During parturition members are entitled to the services of a doctor and a midwife, and to money assistance equal to the basic wage for eight weeks, of which six must be after confinement. There is also, during twelve weeks after the expiration of the benefit just named, a benefit of from one-fifth to half a zloty a day for nursing mothers. If desired, hospital treatment, or home treatment with the attendance of a nurse, may be substituted for the above benefits, the pecuniary benefit being then reduced by one-half.

In case of death there is a grant for funeral expenses, equal to twenty-one times the daily wage of the insured person.

The members of the family of the insured are entitled to the following benefits, if they live in the same household and are dependent on the earnings of the insured:—

(a) Medical attendance or hospital treatment for thirteen weeks.
(b) Maternity assistance without money benefits.
(c) Nursing mothers' benefits, equal to one-half the benefits for insured persons.
(d) Funeral benefits on the same scale as (c).

Certain supplementary benefits are given for insured and their dependents if the reserves of the sickness funds allow of this.

The organisation of each sickness fund is distributed between the board of governors, the managing committee, the supervisory committee, and the board of arbitration.

The board of governors is elected for two-thirds of its members by the insured and for one-third by the employers on the principle of proportional representation. The board elects the managing committee with the same proportion of representatives of the insured and of employers as are maintained on the board.

The supervisory committee is elected each year in a similar way. The board of arbitration settles disputes, and its decisions are final. It consists of two representatives of insured and employers respectively, and one representative of the board of governors as a whole.

Disputes with Doctors.—In each fund's area are special committees for settling these, consisting of representatives of the managing committee and the doctors, with a neutral chairman nominated by both parties.

For certain common duties regional unions of funds are formed, and these again combine in one general union of funds. These carry on institutional, statistical, and other work which can be done co-operatively.

The State supervises from two departments: from the Ministry of Labour and Social Welfare for general administration, and from the Ministry of the Interior (General Directorate of the Public Health Service) for medical matters. Each of these ministries nominates representatives to the staff of each insurance office.

For further legal and other particulars, *Social Insurance in Poland*, by Francois Sokal, Minister of Labour and Social Welfare (Geneva, 1925), should be consulted.

Number Insured.—At the beginning of 1925, 1,883,905 were insured for sickness, or 4,173,000 including their families. This total is equal to 15·5 per cent. of the total population of Poland. At that time, of the total 161 sickness funds—

> 31 had less than 2,000 members,
> 45 had 2,000–5,000 members,
> 58 had 5,000–10,000 members,
> 21 had 10,000–30,000 members, and
> 6 had more than this number of members.

The proportion of the population which is insured has steadily increased. Thus in Warsaw at the present time 471,000 (including families) are insured, or about half of the total population; and this is true also for Posen.

Arrangements for Medical Aid.—In the former Prussian territories, in which German sickness insurance existed before the Great War, unlimited choice of doctor by the insured has been retained. No general rule on this point is laid down by the new Act of 1920, but the system of giving medical aid at dispensaries (ambulatories) specially organised by the funds has been most often adopted. This is the system in Warsaw. Bedridden patients are seen at home by the medical officer of the fund; and the area of each fund is divided into districts, each served by regional medical officers. These visits may be only diagnostic, the doctor then deciding whether home treatment shall be continued or the patient sent to a general or special hospital. The doctor can call in a specialist if he desires.

In the year 1924, according to Sokal (*op. cit.*, p. 74), the number of dispensary consultations was ten times the number of domiciliary visits in Poland as a whole.

For particulars as to the insurance organisation in Warsaw I am greatly indebted to Dr. Wroczynski, former head of the public health work in Warsaw, now in temporary charge of its insurance work. For any comments on parts of this work I am alone responsible.

The entire system of sickness insurance appears to me to have been too rapidly improvised, and it bears evidence of its hasty establishment in nearly all respects. Doubtless this hasty improvisation was owing in part to the need to take up and extend the already existing insurance systems. In this respect one is reminded of the current experience of France, which is undertaking a general system of compulsory sickness insurance, Alsace-Lorraine having such a system already, inherited from its German past (see p. 90). It seems likely that in Poland, Czecho-Slovakia, Hungary, and Austria another motive has been operative in the rapid extension of social insurance, viz. that thus each worker would have a stake in social stability and a bulwark would be raised against the extension of Bolshevism.

One of the great difficulties in sickness insurance in Poland—elsewhere also in some measure—is the lack of general appreciation of its true character, insured persons commonly wanting an almost immediate return for their payments.

Other difficulties and drawbacks will be gathered from the following notes. Notwithstanding, it must be agreed that, apart from insurance for medical attendance, the social and hygienic position of the population of Poland and the economic position of its doctors would be immensely worse than it actually is, in view of the extreme poverty which prevails. The too small number of doctors are made more generally available under insurance than would otherwise be possible, even if there were less financial stress than actually exists.

The relation of insurance medical work to the work of the municipal and State hospitals is not satisfactory. The hospital beds are inadequate for the national needs; and much dissatisfaction is expressed by city and district local authorities because they are only paid one-half of the expenditure incurred in treating insured patients. This will probably be readjusted ere long.

In Warsaw only 80 hospital beds have been specially provided for insured patients by the sickness funds. Other hospitals are municipal or private. There are altogether some 5,000 hospital beds, but this is inadequate. I heard of a patient being sent to as many as nine hospitals before he secured a bed.

The city hospitals are used for maternity cases. Of the 7,500 confinements among the insured in one year in Warsaw, most are attended by midwives, but in nearly one-third a doctor is also called in.

In 1928 new regulations for *midwives* were issued by the Government, which, as possibilities of training midwives increase, should lead to a great improvement in the present unsatisfactory position of this work.

The *ambulatories* in Warsaw, which are the chief centres for treatment, have very few good dispensary buildings. Very often private houses have been taken, and their small corridors are crowded for hours with patients awaiting treatment. This may be expected to be improved gradually; but, as in other countries, it appeared to me that the ambulatory system, unless skilfully organised and constantly supervised from this point of view, must continue to mean an inordinate waste of time for the patient, if not also a feeling on the part of the doctor that he must hurry to receive the next patient, which is detrimental to good clinical work.

The worst feature of the ambulatories is the uncontrolled access of insured patients to any doctor they may select. Fifty per cent. of the patients who attend the eight larger ambulatories in Warsaw never come back for a second consultation. This is absolutely inimical to good diagnosis and treatment. There is no continuity of medical supervision and responsibility, without which medical advice is largely wasted. A patient sometimes goes on the same day to several clinics. The ability to "follow up" patients may be regarded as the basis of preventive medicine as applied to personal medical practice. How to secure it in the treatment of patients on a large scale is a pressing problem of insurance medical practice, not merely in Poland, but throughout Western Europe.

The free choice of doctors at the ambulatories precludes

any accurate registration of cases on cards or otherwise. It is a system of specialism, the patient choosing which so-called specialist he will see.

There is now some regulation of the number of patients a doctor may see per hour. It is limited to six for most cases; dentists may see only four in the hour; oculists may see ten.

In Warsaw doctors are paid at the rate of 8·70 zlotys per hour of medical work either at the ambulatory or in home treatment. In 1928, in the Warsaw ambulatories, there were 2,880,000 medical consultations.

Warsaw is divided for insurance work into 200 districts, doctors not chosen by the patient making home visits as required. The choice of doctors is made in one of the eight large ambulatories in Warsaw. An instance was quoted to me of ten physicians visiting a particular patient within fifteen days. In winter there are not enough insurance doctors for the work required; and in one influenza epidemic 400 additional temporary doctors were engaged. There are 2,200 doctors in Warsaw; evidently the present permanent staff of 200 for domiciliary work must be increased. There is a special organisation for seeing urgent cases. At first this was confined to obstetric and gynæcological cases. It is said now to be much abused.

I ascertained that there was excessive prescribing of drugs, similar to what is experienced in other national insurance schemes. A medical committee has investigated this, and it may be hoped that in time treatment will become more hygienic and less empirical.

The question as to the *number of doctors* employed by the insurance funds is one of great difficulty. Doctors are only placed on the staff when accepted by the Medical Union of Warsaw. At present there are 800 doctors in Warsaw awaiting insurance appointments. As doctors are paid by the hour, it is evident that increase of staff would imply a lower average income for each doctor. Thus the medical profession is divided on this essential point.

There is much discussion as to the methods of treatment

of insured patients and as to the best methods for reform, the need for which is generally accepted. The present excessive use of the consultation arrangements at ambulatories is, in my view, the root of the evil. It is contrary to the interest of patients themselves that there should be *no doctor whom each insured patient can claim as his own*, and from whom he can secure treatment which is based on accurate diagnosis of present illness conjoined with a knowledge of the patient's past history, and so far as practicable of the history of his family.

The need for expert consultations will remain; but the lack of close relation of these to the work of the general practitioner is a serious defect in present conditions. Present arrangements in Warsaw appeared to me both extravagant and inefficient, and will, I think, lead to bankruptcy of insurance funds if not made more efficient, and thus more economical.

I should at this point express my indebtedness to Dr. E. Piestrzynski, through whose courtesy I had during my stay in Warsaw the daily help of Dr. S. Tubiasz of the Department of Public Health in the Ministry of the Interior. Dr. Tubiasz rendered me invaluable service. He arranged a conference with representatives of the medical profession in Warsaw, and his linguistic skill enabled one to obtain a clear view of the professional attitude of doctors to the Polish sickness insurance system. Those who took part in this conference were :—

(*a*) Dr. Zamecki Stanislaw, President of the Warsaw Branch of the Polish Medical Union.

(*b*) Dr. Adam Przyborowski, former President of the Medical Chamber of Warsaw.

(*c*) Dr. Waetan Stefanski, Chairman of the Committee for Health Insurance Problems at the P.M. Union.

(*d*) Dr. Jan Zaluska, General Secretary of Polish Medical Union.

It was made clear at this conference that the medical profession in Poland are not opposed to the principle of sickness insurance, though they object to some of the actual methods employed. They regard it as impossible to abolish sickness insurance, but they require certain modifications which will make the medical working of the scheme compatible with the dignity and welfare of the medical profession.

After a valuable interview, it was arranged that I should write to Dr. Zaluska, and that the Medical Union would then send me a considered statement as to their attitude, not only to sickness insurance, but also to certain medical activities of public health authorities.

I append the correspondence embodying this arrangement. It does not appear to me to call for special comment; I consider myself fortunate in having elicited this authoritative statement of the attitude and desires of the Polish medical profession.

The questions submitted by me were the following:—

1. Whether the conditions of medical work at present are satisfactory as regards payment by hours of work.

2. Whether any system of payment by number of insured persons enrolled on the doctors' list would be preferred.

3. Whether it would be well to extend domiciliary treatment of patients and limit the visits to the ambulatories.

4. Whether the wandering of patients from doctor to doctor should be limited.

5. Whether, as a result of the above, there should be some limitation of free choice as well as of change of doctors.

6. Should any action be taken to restrict excessive prescription of drugs, if this be possible?

7. Is any restriction of the excessive use of present expert consultative facilities desirable?

8. Whether any further lines of action are possible which will enable the doctors to assist in economising the funds of insurance, an object by which doctors would themselves secure an improved financial status.

9. Should there be any limitation to gratuitous attendance of tuberculous and venereal patients at clinics at the public expense?

STATEMENT

WARSAW,
July 27, 1929.

DEAR SIR ARTHUR NEWSHOLME,
Your letter of May 26th has been handed to us for attention by Dr. Zaluska, secretary of the Zw.L.P.P. The points brought up by you have been the subject of discussions at our meetings of the Executive Committee, and the replies we furnish can be considered as the official opinions of the officers of the Zw.L.P.P. as to the questions brought up by you.

We desire first of all to inform you that in Poland we have not yet in existence a uniform system of affording medical help to those insured against illness; thus in certain districts the ambulatory system is in force, in certain others the system of free choice of medical advice—the so-called panel system—and finally the mixed system also holds good in a number of localities.

We beg to answer the questions propounded by you in the same order, viz. :—

1. Conditions of medical work are hardly satisfactory in so far as payment by hours of work is applied. Physicians are paid from 6–8 zlotys per hour of consultation: thus even working five hours a day the average monthly salary earned is between 750–1,000 zlotys. This cannot be considered as sufficient, especially for highly-qualified and older doctors.

2. The system of payment by number of insured on doctor's list has not been tried in Poland, and, having no experience of this mode in practice, we cannot offer any concrete opinion. For that matter, this system can be applied only in those cases where the panel system is in force: it cannot be applied where the ambulatory system is issued, nor in larger cities where the inhabitants are used to being cured by specialists. Under certain conditions, it would seem that this system should be tried out.

3. The question of extending domiciliary treatment and restricting ambulatory methods is covered by the preceding reply.

4. The wandering of patients from doctor to doctor should be restricted. This is sufficiently foreseen and allowed for in the Polish Health Insurance Act.

5. The limitation of free choice of doctors by patients is not indicated. With regard to wandering from doctor to doctor, this should be controlled as regards the utility of such wandering by medical organisations.

6. Action to be taken for the restricting of excessive prescription of drugs is essential and should be directed in two directions: (*a*) influencing the doctors to prescribe the simplest medicines possible recognised by the medical profession, and (*b*) charging the patient with a certain percentage of the cost of the medicine.

7. The question of the desirability of the restriction of excessive use of expert consultative facilities is covered by our answers to questions 4 and 5.

8. Further lines of action along which doctors could assist in economising the funds of insurance necessarily exist, and such co-operation should be carried out. Such would be for example:—

(*a*) Health propaganda and instruction amongst patients.

(*b*) Combating of simulation and dishonest practices.

(*c*) Economy in the use of drugs.

(*d*) Rational certifying of unfitness to work.

(*e*) In general economy and the rational granting of all services, as also in opposition to excessive demands made by patients.

(*f*) Economies in the actual administration of Health Insurance.

It must be added with regard to the statement that such economies would tend to raise the standard of payment for medical services, that this is not necessarily so in Poland. It is certainly true that the medical profession could aid and bring about economies and prevent wasteful use of the funds. On the other hand, Poland has so many arrears to catch up in the field of hygiene and such an insufficient number of hospitals, sanatoria, etc., that no matter what economies are made, numerous other demands more urgent than those of doctors' salaries would have first call for the money saved. The question of increasing this remuneration of doctors should therefore be treated as entirely independent of any economies effected with or without their aid. For that matter the attainment of higher salaries for doctors as a result of economies effected upon the treatment of the patients would result in the creation of an abnormal situation incompatible and harmful to the interests of the medical profession.

President: DR. FALKOWSKI.
Secretary: DR. J. ZALUSKA.

Posen

The information culled by me in a rather brief visit to Posen is inserted here as supplementing in some aspects the contents of the preceding pages.

Through the kindness of Dr. Schultz, the health officer of this great town, I was placed in touch with Professor Dr. Jonscher, who showed me the important children's clinic and hospital in Posen, of which he is the physician. This is one part of the teaching clinics of the University of Posen.

There are thirty-six beds, and an out-patients' department at which both "well babies" and sick babies are seen daily. At the station for well babies, milk is supplied under regulated conditions. This is one of five or six similar stations in different parts of Posen.

There is accurate registration of births in Posen within three or four days after birth, and the mothers are visited at home by a nurse from the station. The district served from this hospital clinic is small, having a population of only 15,000 to 20,000.

The milk supplied when artificial feeding cannot be avoided is paid for by those who can pay, otherwise by the municipality. Many sick babies are seen and treated, even when the parents are insured.

As in other parts of Poland, the children of insured persons are entitled to treatment by the insurance doctors; but in practice this treatment is said to be limited and unsatisfactory, and is only provided for a maximum period of three months. Thus insured persons and their children often are seen only two or three times if ill, and not throughout an illness. This applies, for instance, to rickets or chronic bronchitis in children. The possibility of such treatment elsewhere is not allowed to interfere with continued satisfactory treatment of sick children at the University clinic. The insurance funds pay the clinic for any specialist diagnosis and treatment required by them (e.g. use of Röntgen rays or quartz lamp); also sometimes for the treatment of in-patients who are children of insured

persons. A main consideration at this clinic is to obtain
adequate cases for medical teaching.

After the consultation for infants, home visits are made
by the nurses to ensure efficiency of home management.

The clinic comprises a department for Calmette vaccination. Cases are specially selected; already 1,500 cases
have been protected. These come from families where there
is a case of open tuberculosis. After vaccination the child
is isolated for three or four weeks, either in the beds
attached to this clinic or in a city hospital. The clinic also
has a preventorium for children from tuberculosis families.
The society for combating tuberculosis partially supports
the work done in this connection.

There are special departments at the clinic for nervous,
cutaneous, and venereal patients. No one is refused, whatever
his income.

From Dr. Wierusz, State District Officer of Health of
the rural communes of Posen and chief medical officer of
its insurance fund, I also received valuable help. His offices
are situate in a large building in Posen, which serves in
respect of both these functions. The combination of officers
and of buildings has been brought about by co-operation
between the rural health authority and the insurance fund
(krankenkasse), the cost of buildings, their maintenance,
and of salaries being shared between the two. One condition of the amalgamation has been that not only shall the
50 per cent. of the population which is insured be treated
in this institution, but others also.

The offices are used as an ambulatorium, in which
Dr. Wierusz and several other doctors see patients not too
ill to attend at a central building. Altogether eight practising physicians co-operate in this joint scheme. For rural
parts there are smaller stations for consultations, at which
also non-insured as well as insured are treated.

Accompanied by Dr. Wierusz, I subsequently saw one
of these rural health centres. This is partly supported by
voluntary contributions, but is subsidised by the insurance
fund. It has a dispensary for infants and for tuberculous

patients, as well as for general medical cases. It is stated that at least 70 per cent. of the total infants of the district are supervised from this centre.

From my inquiries in Posen, as supplementing those made in Warsaw, I give the following particulars, with their associated reflections.

In this division of Poland doctors are paid for attendance on patients per case of illness (not per insured patient on the doctor's panel). The work in this part of Poland is conducted on the "cabinet system", i.e. by home visits and consultations in the doctor's private office. The chief physician to the insurance fund decides whether a consultation is needed for any patient. This means too few consultations: in Warsaw they are excessive in number. Posen, with its population of a quarter of a million, constitutes one insurance fund (krankenkasse). Accounts for work done are sent in every half-year through the committee of the doctors' union, who are expected to vouch for their accuracy, the krankenkasse also employing a physician for revision of accounts.

The doctors' union has entered into a contract with the krankenkasse in virtue of which 18 per cent. of the income from the insured is paid to doctors attending the insured. This is expected to include also payment for the services of specialists. The doctors are not satisfied with this payment; and the details of the system do not appear to be satisfactory. They have, it appears to me, been arranged from the point of view of specialists rather than of medicine as a complete art. There is a system of counting "points" for each case. Thus a general examination will count as two, while a simple injection (as a hypodermic) will count also as two. Or a doctor will charge two points for diagnosis of a doubtful pulmonary case, and two points for an injection. Such marking does not conduce to complete examination of the patient. Points are more easily made by other methods than by a complete all-round diagnosis, and the "points" as at present arranged distort the medical needs of the insured. It has been found possible to make good "points" and to see as many as forty to fifty patients in two hours! For home visits points are allowed for distance.

The 200 doctors in Posen are almost entirely supported by their insurance work. Not more than ten doctors rely on private practice, including the University professors. The population of Posen is regarded by those competent to judge as too large for a single krankenkasse. Both too large and too small districts are bad from the point of view of the insured. The power possessed by the Ministry of Social Welfare to combine insurance funds is not utilised. Supervision of the work in excessively large districts is difficult or impracticable.

I was informed that the insured were not altogether contented with their treatment; dissatisfaction appeared to take chiefly the form of fear that the drugs supplied to them by the official druggists were inferior, and were given by doctors with an eye to cheapness.

More than one physician with whom I conversed referred to the immense financial power of the larger krankenkassen, and especially of the combined funds of the krankenkassen. They exercise immense political influence, for there are large moneys at their disposal, and the control of the Government over them is hesitant and feeble. One physician regarded the insurance funds as a "State within the State" which possessed great possibilities of evil as well as of good.

There are several infant welfare centres and tuberculosis dispensaries in Posen, mostly run by the municipality. There is some medical inspection of school children, but no treatment is undertaken.

A dental cabinet for poor children was started a few months ago by the municipality. Payment is required according to patients' means.

CHAPTER VII

CZECHO-SLOVAKIA[1]

PRELIMINARY SUMMARY

Strenuous and ambitious efforts have been successfully made to place the medico-hygienic organisation of this new country on progressive lines. The training of all health officers has been organised. The medical care of the poor is somewhat hampered by the still inadequate number of trained nurses.

Sickness insurance on compulsory lines will soon include nearly the entire population. It is organised on national lines. As a rule there is no free choice of doctors for the insured. Large central institutes (polyclinics) exist to a possibly excessive extent.

The position of doctors in regard to public medical work is set out by Dr. Helbech for the National Association of Physicians on page 243.

My visit to Prague to inquire into the medico-hygienic provisions of the new republic of Czecho-Slovakia was made pleasant and easy by the active assistance rendered me by some of its chief social workers, to whom my indebtedness is more fully acknowledged in subsequent paragraphs.

The new republic, a product of the Great War, has been carved out of Austria, Germany, and Hungary. Before the war most of its territory belonged to the former Austro-Hungarian Empire, consisting of three parts—Bohemia, Moravia, and Silesia—each with its own administrative system, and representing different standards of civilisation and of organisation.

In general contour it resembles a somewhat swollen fish, the head of which (Bohemia) is surrounded on three sides by Germany, while its middle part is between Poland and the Austrian republic, and its tail is between Poland and

[1] Date of investigation, May–June 1929.

the reduced Hungary. While realising the ideal of an independent Czecho-Slavonic State, it is thus a sort of bridge between Western and Eastern Europe.

It is largely mountainous and has no seaboard, its waters emptying into the North Sea, the Baltic Sea, and the Black Sea. It belongs to the group of Danubian States.

Its population is chiefly agricultural, and it is almost independent of imported food. It has also some well-developed industries. In Bohemia about 30 per cent., in Moravia 41 per cent., in Silesia 29 per cent., and in Slovakia 61 per cent. of the population are engaged in agriculture.

Czecho-Slovakia has an area of about 140,000 square kilometres and a population of about 14 millions, and of this population 65·5 per cent. are of Czech and Slovak, 23·3 per cent. of German, 5·5 per cent. of Magyar, and 3·5 per cent. of Sub-Carpathian Ruthenian origin; while 1·4 per cent. are Jews, and a smaller number of Polish or other origin. The country thus has among its problems that of minority races, the assimilation of which is far from easy. The greater part of the population is Roman Catholic.

GOVERNMENT

The constitution of the Czecho-Slovak republic was adopted in February 1920; and it will be realised, therefore, that in their present form most of its medico-hygienic activities have only recently come into operation.

Its constitution is headed by an elected President. Its national Parliament consists of two chambers: a Chamber of Deputies, consisting of 300 members elected for a period of six years, and a Senate, consisting of 150 members, to be renewed every eight years. The President is elected for a period of seven years by these two bodies sitting in joint session.

The franchise for the Chamber of Deputies is open to all citizens of both sexes who are over 21; the franchise for the Senate is open to all citizens who are over 26.

The responsibility in the Government for medico-hygienic administration is in the hands of the

> Ministry of Health and Physical Education, and
> Ministry of Social Welfare.

Education, which necessarily bears largely on health prospects, is compulsory between the ages of 6 and 14.

The central partition of medico-hygienic work between the two ministries named above means that the national system of insurance against sickness and much of child hygiene work is not centrally guided and controlled by the Ministry of Health. Local administration is in the hands of provincial, communal, and district authorities.

HEALTH ADMINISTRATION IN PRAGUE

The administration of Prague may be cited in illustration of the public health administration of Czecho-Slovakia at its point of maximum efficiency. In making my inquiries in Prague I had the great advantage of being accompanied by Dr. Riha, a medical official of the Ministry of Health, whose efficient services were kindly lent by Dr. Antonin Kolinsky, head of the Ministry of Health. I also received valuable assistance from Dr. Leach, the local representative of the Rockefeller Foundation, and from Drs. Feierabend and H. J. Pelc of the State Hygienic Institute.

Prague has a population of some 700,000. It is divided into twenty-four wards, in one of which (the thirteenth district) is the Health Demonstration mentioned below, which was begun in 1927. This district has a whole-time medical officer, whose salary, as well as a part of the equipment of the health centre, is paid by the Rockefeller Foundation.

Altogether Prague has seventy-two part-time health officers under a chief M.O.H., who is a whole-time officer. These officers not only carry out local work for the control of epidemics, etc., but also verify the causes of death—acting as coroners—and make school medical inspections to the small extent that this work is done outside the demonstration area.

TRAINING OF HEALTH OFFICERS

All these officers are required to pass their *physikat*,[1] which is similar in some respects to the English diploma in public health. Any doctor can be admitted to this examination after having been two years engaged as resident in a hospital or three years in private practice. No special curriculum is demanded, though a non-official three months' course is given at the University in preparation for the physikat.

Under a new scheme now being initiated, in which the Hygienic Institute and the University are co-operating, a six months' curriculum will be demanded from every candidate for the post of health officer.

Outside Prague, rural doctors find it difficult to earn a living wage unless they hold the position of part-time health officer. The health officers for small rural districts are appointed by the State.

SPECIAL DEMONSTRATION DISTRICT

The Special Demonstration District of Prague has been organised by joint effort of the City Council, the Rockefeller Foundation, and a number of voluntary organisations. This district has a population of about 46,000, of which three-fourths are urban and one-fourth rural in character. The population consists chiefly of weekly wage-earners and small officials, tenement houses being the rule.

In its health centre are focussed all the health activities of the district, subject to a satisfactory liaison with the general city organisation. In it all the work of collecting local vital statistics is carried out, of controlling infectious diseases, of school medical inspection, industrial hygiene, and housing. Here also are held clinics for tuberculosis and venereal disease, and consultations for mothers and young children; and the social assistance bureau of the district is in the same building. Special attention may be called to this placing of machinery for investigation of poverty and

[1] An abbreviation of physikat examination. The old name for the chief medical officer of the country was Kreisfysicus; hence fysicat examination.

for help in kind in close conjunction with the medico-hygienic agencies.

The total cost of the demonstration is borne to the extent of four-fifths by the city and one-fifth from various voluntary sources. It has five public health nurses and a supervisor in addition to its whole-time health officers, and four part-time physicians for each of the consultations named above and for school work.

Every birth is notified, and visits at home are made within a week. In this district about one-half of the total infants are kept under supervision until they reach school age.

An obstetrician holds an antenatal clinic weekly at the health centre. Much active work has been done in immunisation of children against diphtheria.

There has been arranged a permanent federation of all private health and social agencies in the demonstration area.

The public health nursing in the area has been organised on a generalised plan, each of the five nurses undertaking complete responsibility for a particular sub-district.

There is close co-operation in the area with the official insurance organisation. As most of the population are insured for medical treatment, the giving of medical advice at the health centre seldom needs to be supplemented by treatment.

School medical inspection in the demonstration area is thorough. Much dental treatment is carried out gratuitously in the cases in which the needed treatment cannot be secured through insurance channels.

No difficulty has been experienced with private medical practitioners, as nearly the entire population is insured, and insurance doctors are not paid per attendance.

In the special area each child is examined thoroughly on entering school; and every child is again thoroughly examined before leaving school, and occupational guidance given.

The school doctor visits each school in his own area quarterly, special children being picked out for him by the teacher or nurse. In the special area each assistant medical officer functions as—

School doctor,
Doctor for all who cannot otherwise secure treatment,
Doctor for the control of infectious diseases, and
Certifier of causes of death in the district.

A somewhat novel activity of the demonstration area is the

Anti-Alcoholic Clinic

During 1928, 117 alcoholics attended at this special clinic, making 408 attendances. Some 1,162 visits were made at the homes of these alcoholics. The clinic is conducted by a group of social workers, one of whom is a psychiatrist. Patients are derived from several sources. Some names are given by the police from among persons arrested for drunkenness. These are invited to attend on a particular day, and some come, as shown above. An informal collective talk follows, and then a promise to abstain for a week is asked. Five or six promises may be obtained from twenty present. The family is visited, and the co-operation of the wife is sought. Those who abstain for three months are regarded as having graduated, and some of these reformed alcoholics volunteer to co-operate in visiting other alcoholics.

Sometimes applications for help are received directly from the relatives of the addict.

Similar institutions in Warsaw and Vienna have had considerable success.

There is active propagandism in favour of alcoholic abstinence throughout Czecho-Slovakia; and in Sub-Carpathian Ruthenia the State has given a special subsidy in aid of propagandist literature in the Ruthenian and Hungarian languages.

State Hygienic Institute

The progress of hygiene in Czecho-Slovakia has been helped and accelerated by the State Institute of Hygiene in Prague, in the initiation of which the Rockefeller Foundation has taken an important part. To this will be added shortly a large expansion of the institute on the social side of hygiene, along with a School of Public Health and Hygiene. To Dr. Feierabend, the vice-director of the institute, and to Dr. Pelc, the head of its social hygiene division, I am much indebted for the help they rendered me.

The State Hygienic Institute is in fact a part of the Ministry of Health, carrying out for the Ministry important functions in diagnosis of disease, and in the production, supervision, and standardisation of sera and vaccines and of pharmaceutical preparations; also in the examination of water and sewage. Throughout its organisation, although the work is thoroughly scientific, research is made secondary to immediate practical utility in administration.

At the institute last year some 1,600,000 individual supplies of smallpox vaccine lymph were sent out to health officers throughout the country gratuitously, the State bearing the expense.

In Prague there are four branch diagnostic laboratories attached to the institute, and others in some provincial areas. No national settlement has been made as to payment for these examinations, but material sent by health officers is examined free of charge. Private practitioners are expected to pay for specimens sent when their patients can afford this. For insurance patients the insurance organisation pays. These limitations must have some inhibitory influence in the needed diagnosis of syphilis, tuberculosis, etc.

On its social hygiene side the Hygienic Institute is only now in process of full development. This side will have a research division, including field work in selected areas, and will be devoted largely to health propaganda and definite educational work. The instruction to be given will include, among others, special courses for public health officers, public health nurses, and others engaged in public health work. This division of the institute will absorb the School of Social Work, in which at present thirty pupils are trained for public health and social work in a two years' course.

NURSES

A great need of Czecho-Slovakia is a rapid increase in the number of skilled nurses, both for the sick in hospitals and for public health work. Half the nurses in hospitals are inadequately trained members of religious orders. This need will have to be met if the population are within the next few years to be brought to appreciate the importance and value of health measures.

MEDICAL CARE OF POOR

Much social work of importance is being done by the city of Prague in Dr. Zenkl's department of the city administration dealing with social welfare (Prévoyance Social). This department has taken the place of what would correspond to our care of paupers, the use of any similar word being tabooed. A large staff of women are engaged in investigating cases of destitution and in recommending appropriate measures. In Dr. Zenkl's words: "Official efforts formerly taken to relieve or remove pauperism were stamped by a spirit of condescendence entirely conven-tional." This has now been replaced by "Research into the ills of society, not only with a view to palliation or recovery, but also in order to remove their causes".

The measures taken in fulfilment of this ideal are not dissimilar from those of other communities. For carrying them out, as elsewhere, a skilled social investigator is needed, somewhat above the standard of the rural "relieving officer" in England, and one not bound down by legal conditions which preclude help prior to the actual state of destitution. But in Prague, as in other cities, the measures taken to help the impoverished need to be more intimately related to the medical and hygienic work of the public health authority.

When monetary relief is directly required, there is justification for a special staff to investigate the conditions of giving this; but a *caveat* (not specially applicable to one country, but of general significance) may be entered as to the doubtful desirability of dual visiting in the homes of the poor by public health visitors and by social workers, when there is no immediate question of destitution. As a rule the public health nurse, if well trained, is quite competent to report on both hygienic and social needs and to give the needed advice in the home and to her official employers.

MIDWIFERY

Midwifery in Czecho-Slovakia is chiefly in the hands of midwives, who attend nearly all the births. Every midwife must have undergone a five or six months' course of training in one of the five midwifery schools in the country. Proposals are on foot to extend the training and to secure a better distribution of midwives. As a rule the number in country districts is inadequate.

NATIONAL COUNCIL OF SOCIAL HYGIENE

Under this council, of which Dr. Alice Masaryk is the president, the activities of the Red Cross, of the Masaryk League against Tuberculosis, of the Association for Combating Venereal Diseases, of the Maternity and Welfare Association, and of the Temperance Association have been federated. By this means overlapping of efforts is minimised, and it has become possible to make a joint appeal for funds.

It is unnecessary for our purpose to describe in detail the activities of the different societies enumerated above. These are indicated by their titles.

The Masaryk League against Tuberculosis has as its main activity the formation of anti-tuberculosis dispensaries of which there are now about 200 in the country. At an earlier stage the doctors in charge of these dispensaries, as also of child-welfare stations and dispensaries for venereal diseases, undertook the treatment of the patients attending the dispensaries. This determined some measure of hostility in the minds of doctors engaged in private practice; but, especially at tuberculosis dispensaries, the physicians now limit their activities in the main to diagnosis and hygienic advice, and relations have improved.

Dr. Helbech, the secretary of the Medical Association in Prague, informed me that these dispensaries now limited themselves to preventive work. In Slovakia, however, it has been found necessary to treat patients at the dispensaries; otherwise they will not attend (see also page 245).

The death-rate from tuberculosis in Czecho-Slovakia is excessive. In Dr. J. Hrdlička's contribution to the *Annuaire Sanitaire Internationale*, 1925 (Société des Nations), it is stated that in 1925 pulmonary tuberculosis was the cause of death of 17·2 and tuberculosis of other organs of 2·1 per 10,000 inhabitants. This high death-rate is much lower than that in the pre-war period.

VENEREAL DISEASES

This subject has been fully treated in a brochure by Dr. H. J. Pelc,[1] and from this and long conversations with Dr. Pelc the following summary of the subject is derived.

The law governing action was passed in 1922. This made it obligatory on any person suffering from a venereal disease to undergo treatment by a duly licensed physician. Suspected cases (subject to safeguardings of the good reputation of the person concerned!) may be examined compulsorily by order of the Board of Health; and in some circumstances compulsory treatment in an institution can be enforced. Physicians must notify if the patient neglects treatment.

The law has not been effective. There has been difficulty, arising from doubt as to the relative functions of the Ministries of Health and of Social Welfare in its administration, especially as regards prostitutes. Difficulty has also arisen in the provision of treatment. The resort to venereal disease dispensaries has been disappointingly scanty. Indigent patients are treated gratuitously. For others the

[1] *On Venereal Diseases in the Czecho-Slovak Republic*, by Dr. Hynek J. Pelc. With 59 tables and 40 diagrams.

machinery enabling a supply of a salvarsan preparation to be obtained is almost prohibitive. In Prague even indigent patients have to be sent to a special office to obtain salvarsan, which they then take back to the clinic! In rural districts a direct application must be made to the Minister of Health for salvarsan. This was doubtless dictated by motives of economy, but in practice it means the avoidable persistence of rampant disabling disease.

In the province of Slovakia, however, salvarsan is supplied gratuitously.

The problem is modified by the fact that so large a proportion of the total population is insured. As shown in the following pages, there is both sickness and invalidity insurance. Treatment of venereal disease under the sickness insurance system does not work well in rural districts, and not very well even in towns. The tendency is for the patient to be treated only so long as symptoms persist, in part because the insurance doctor has no special incentive to press for continued treatment and to educate his patient to this end.

But it is becoming recognised that venereal diseases are a great cause of chronic and premature invalidity; and there is little doubt that with increasing realisation of this serious economic fact there will be further organised effort to diminish this serious drain on the funds of invalidity insurance by adequate treatment.

SICKNESS INSURANCE

The political history of Czecho-Slovakia since its formation in 1920 is one of almost feverish activity to promote social welfare. This is the most characteristic feature of its legislation during its short history; and it would appear that the brave and impressive efforts already made would have been still greater but for the hampering of financial stress.

The Republic took over from former Austria the accident and sickness insurance for industrial workers and the pension system for private officials; and a colossal building in Prague now houses the administrative centre for the national pension scheme for employees in private concerns.

The particulars of the national scheme for accident and for unemployment insurance need not further concern us here.

In 1924 a new general and compulsory insurance of all employees for invalidity and old age, for sickness, and for unemployment was enacted; and by this law the way was also prepared for a prospective insurance of all independent workers, i.e. those not employed for wage or salary. This portion of the national insurance scheme has not been carried out. The difficulty of collecting contributions seems to be insuperable.

The completion of this scheme means that nearly the entire population will insure benefits in sickness, invalidity, and old age. The organisation and finance of the insurance of independent workers is kept separate from that for employees.

At the time of this national enactment there already existed many separate sickness insurance organisations. These have been continued; the administration of insurance against invalidity and old age, however, being entirely centralised, but with the proviso that there must be co-operation in medical matters. The essential need of this is evident, as otherwise (and even now to some extent) there is a constant tendency to shift the burden of persistent sickness on to the finance of invalidity insurance. It is becoming better appreciated that the burden of invalidity insurance and of premature old age may be diminished by competent medical aid at an earlier stage (page 238).

For sickness insurance there are the following categories of insurance societies:—

1. District insurance institutions, comprising in 1925 71·5 per cent. of the total insured.
2. District agricultural institutions, comprising in 1925 4·6 per cent. of the total insured.

3. Industrial and occupational institutions, comprising in 1925 8·8 per. cent. of the total insured.
4. Professional institutions, comprising in 1925 5·2 per cent. of the total insured.
5. Other institutions, comprising in 1925 9·9 per cent. of the total insured.

The first-named organisations are required to be formed in every political district, and to them, as seen above, most of the insured belong.

The number of persons insured against sickness in 441 insurance societies (caisses) number about 3½ millions, not including some 4 million members of the families of the insured, to whom medical and certain other benefits accrue.

The number falling sick during a recent year was as low as 36·5 per 100 members among agriculturists. It averaged 48·7 for all the insured.

Sickness entitles to a weekly allowance for a period, which may extend to a year, of about 67 per cent. of the weekly earnings of the sick person. The amount paid is about the same proportion to total wages in each of the ten classes into which workers are divided according to wages.

The weekly payment exacted for these benefits generally amounts to 6 per cent. of the insured's pay; very rarely it amounts to 8 per cent. An equal contribution is required from the employer of the insured person.

In addition to the weekly monetary benefit in sickness, the following benefits are given:—

1. Gratuitous attendance in illness, including hospital treatment when necessary for the insured and his family.

2. Maternity benefits. These include the free service of a midwife, and when necessary of a doctor; a monetary allowance the same as in sickness for six weeks before and after confinement if the mother does not undertake paid work in this period and if she is not already personally entitled to sickness benefit; also an additional allowance equal to half the sickness benefit for twelve weeks if she nurses her infant. These benefits apply also to miscarriages.

3. Allowances towards funeral expenses of the insured or his family.

The Quality of Medical Attendance.—There is, as a rule, no free choice of doctors by the insured, though this is allowed in insurance associations for private employees and in farmers' insurance associations. Most insurance societies contract with doctors to attend patients in a given area on a salary or on a *per capita* basis.

In Prague, and in some other towns, a large part of the treatment of the insured is undertaken at a large central institute. I visited the institute at Prague, an enormous building; and Dr. Riha and I were courteously shown every department of its work by Dr. Záhorský, the medical superintendent.

Every need of medicine, including surgery and gynæcology, is provided. Specialists attend for several hours daily; and patients attended by district doctors have the right to consult any of these specialists, independently of the district insurance doctors, if they desire this. Nothing could be more complete or elaborate than the arrangements provided. They include dental treatment, X-ray installations, considerable surgery, various medical baths, and ordinary gratuitous baths for members.

I formed the impression that too much waiting for consultations sometimes occurred; but there could be no doubt as to the high quality of the treatment—without limitation—which was available.

I also gathered the impression that such a large institution, with its elaborate bureaucracy, was necessarily unwieldy, and that—were politics withdrawn—even more efficient, and certainly more economical, arrangements would be practicable.

The unrestrained access of all the insured in Prague to the expert services of this institute must mean a large and unnecessary—and therefore wasteful—use of consultant services, when more judicious selection would have reduced expense and made treatment more efficient and without inordinate delay. Sickness insurance in Czecho-Slovakia, as in Germany, is closely bound up with politics. This is shown in the non-medical appointments at the institutes. A vast financial interest is involved in the insurance funds, and only a constant adherence to financial rigidity and integrity can prevent serious abuses.

The treatment in these institutes is doubtless efficient, but it loses something in the slackening of the personal relationship between patient and doctor. For a vast proportion of the insured, who in the absence of insurance provision would have had no confidential doctor, the medical gain is overwhelming.

There is another difficulty almost always inherent in sickness insurance. It too often serves as an alternative to unemployment insurance. I was told of many workers in the building trades in Prague who, at the end of the season, go to their village homes and at once "go on their club" for sickness insurance benefits.

The question arises—I do not propose to answer it here—as to whether sickness insurance should not be limited to the "socially weak", those for whom no other provision is possible.

Mention may be made in conclusion of the professional classes in Czecho-Slovakia. These are insured for medical attendance, including dental care. I was informed, however, that when the doctor recommended dentures the elaborate system of check and counter-check before the prescription was followed angered the insured persons so much that they often preferred not to avail themselves of the benefit to which they were entitled.

Relation between Official and Private Medical Work.—Some remarks on this have been already made. The conditions as regards insurance medical work are not altogether satisfactory, in part owing to the unwieldy overgrowth of the ambulatory system. As regards other aspects of the problem of interrelation, I have been fortunate in securing the valuable statement specially prepared for me on behalf of the Association of Physicians which follows :—

STATEMENT KINDLY CONTRIBUTED BY THE ASSOCIATION OF PHYSICIANS

I. *Relation between Practising Physicians and School Medical Work—School Doctors*

In our country there are no school clinics where the school children would be treated. In some of our schools—in Greater Prague only—special rooms are provided for school medical work, but they are used and equipped for physical examination of the school children only, and no treatment is given there. Whenever a special examination is necessary which cannot be made by the school doctor—X-rays examination, ophthalmoscopic examination of eyes, etc.—notice is given to the parents or guardians of the child recommending special examination by a röntgenologist, occulist, etc.—no name of specialist being given in the notice. When by an examination of social conditions of the family it is found that it is not possible for the parents of the child to consult a private diagnostician, a special examination is arranged in ambulatories of the appropriate insurance company or in the clinics of the University, or in dispensaries equipped with the necessary outfit for microscopical or X-rays examination.

School children found to be suffering from some disease or physical defect are always referred to a private medical practitioner or specialist; in the family the subject of sickness insurance to the doctor of the sickness insurance company. Indigent cases without sickness insurance are referred to the clinics of the University, where they can be treated without expense.

The slip used for this reference is an official form signed by the school doctor, reads as follows:—

(To be sent in a closed envelope.)

(Date.)

The Report of the Result of the Medical Examination

By the medical examination it was found that your child
. . . .
suffers from . . . .
and it is recommended therefore . . . .

Signature :

City School Doctor

NOTE.—You are kindly requested to state on this slip what measures you took on the strength of this report, then to sign the slip and to return it to the undersigned.

Only children suffering from minor ailments are recommended to the health centres for children, or a choice is given either to see the family doctor or to attend the health centre.

In the years 1909–24 151,355 school children were examined in the elementary schools of Prague. 11,984 of them found to be suffering from disease were referred to the private or insurance doctors. In the schools of Demonstration District—Prague XIIIth—962 children were examined in the last six months, and 291 of them referred to private physicians for treatment.

In view of the law prohibiting school doctors from treating school children in the schools, there are no disputes between the practising physicians and the school medical officers.

Up to this day we have no special school nurses, and no infringement of the rights of practitioners arises from them.

II. *Relation between Practising Physicians and Health Centres*

Our infant centres and dispensaries function now as purely and exclusively preventive prophylactic stations.

In the beginning of their existence—in the war and close post-war time—they could not refuse people asking to be treated. Up to that time the people knew only the curative institutions—ambulatories—and did not comprehend that the new "consulting stations" would follow another idea than that of treatment. Preventive medicine was not a popular science at that time. It appeared to be necessary to instruct the people about the special mission of the health centres, to inform the public about the importance of the preservation of health, periodical examinations of children, etc., and therefore our health centres did not hesitate to care for the sick people like other curative institutions. Six to ten years ago all the dispensaries used to give specific tuberculin treatment—fashionable at that time—to their patients, and many of them developed this treatment at the expense of prevention and education. Later on all of them learned to take care of consumptives for the purpose only of keeping record of them, of getting opportunity to enter their family, their house, and to introduce a proper sanitation in their home and life.

In 1927 our Ministry of Health issued "Regulations on conducting dispensaries". On page 4 of those regulations treatment of tuberculosis patients in the dispensary, as a routine practice, is prohibited.

The anti-tuberculosis dispensary does not attend, as a rule, to the proper curative care. An exception is possible for such persons as were either sent to the dispensary by their attending physician for special—specific—care or those for whom a special treatment could not be provided in another way—indigent people not belonging to a sickness insurance society.

The so-called preventive care—liniments, ultraviolet rays, treatment, etc.—which has for its object to strengthen the resistance of children threatened with tuberculosis, is not classified as proper curative care, and may therefore be given by the dispensary—(paragraph. 4, chapter 2 of the said regulations).

Since that time any encroachment into curative medicine and on the rights of curative physicians on the part of the dispensaries disappeared.

Infant centres were in the same position: they started their work among the people of lower classes, and they had to devote their attention even to sick children, where no other provision for treatment was made. Now, when the comprehension of the necessity of preventive examinations is broadly extended among the public, they give up all curative methods and follow their main function of supervision of the healthy infant and education of the mother. Where treatment is given, it is incidental only—first-aid treatment—and intended to remove some temporary minor ailment for which a well-to-do mother would not think it necessary to call a doctor. Few, if any, drugs, other than those which are nutritive rather than medicinal—e.g. cod-liver oil, etc.—are stocked and dispensed. There is no giving of prescriptions in the health centres. Only cases referred by doctors to be treated in centres—indigent cases—are treated.

In twenty-one children health centres called "Poradny naším dětem"—"Consulting Stations for our Children"—there were 126,799 children examined in regular periodical examinations last year—1928—1,551 of them, being found sick, have been referred to private doctors, 4,927 to the physicians of various insurance companies, and 3,438 to various ambulatories for treatment.

Under these conditions there is no reason for any rivalry between practising physicians and infant consultation centres.

The only clinics where treatment of the patients takes place are the venereal diseases centres, but the persons treated there are of such a kind that there is little hope that they would look after proper treatment in any other way.

The anti-alcoholic clinic operating in Prague XIIIth is also a curative institution: its function is psychotherapeutic treatment of chronic alcoholics referred by the police.

An active co-operation of practising physicians with the health centres, which would consist in notifying cases in need of preventive care and referring such cases to the health centres, is very rare so far as the children, prenatal, venereal, and other clinics are concerned; more often it can be noted with tuberculosis clinics.

Dr. B. Helbech,

Director of the Public Health Demonstration in Prague XIIIth,
and Secretary of the Association of Physicians.

Prague,
   June 1, 1929.

INDEX

[*See also Table of Contents, page* 15]